Side Effects

*A Nurse's Journey Through
Secondary Traumatic Stress*

D.B. WRIGHT

◆ FriesenPress

Suite 300 - 990 Fort St
Victoria, BC, V8V 3K2
Canada

www.friesenpress.com

Copyright © 2016 D.B. Wright
First Edition — 2016

Author Photo by Colleen Serban Photography.
Cover image designed by Andrew Ostrovsky.

All rights reserved.

Disclaimer: The names of patients, nurses and doctors have been changed to maintain their confidentiality.

No part of this publication may be reproduced in any form, or by any means, electronic or mechanical, including photocopying, recording, or any information browsing, storage, or retrieval system, without permission in writing from FriesenPress.

ISBN
978-1-4602-9190-0 (Hardcover)
978-1-4602-9191-7 (Paperback)
978-1-4602-9192-4 (eBook)

1. BIOGRAPHY & AUTOBIOGRAPHY, MEDICAL

Distributed to the trade by The Ingram Book Company

This book is dedicated to all those who witness the suffering of others.

Part One
2005–2006

The journey of a thousand miles
begins with one step.
—Lao Tzu

Chapter 1

He was flatline when they brought him in. CPR in progress as they wheeled him in on a stretcher, a large flap of his scalp being held in place by a hastily applied gauze.

"Seventeen-year-old male in an MVA. Right front passenger, belted, car broadsided from the right. Vital signs absent."

The physician looks over at me. "Okay guys, let's get to work and save a life."

Only we didn't save him. As if it were yesterday, I feel myself tense. Every nerve ending in my body has fired up in preparation for action. Usually the way this goes is I spend the next several minutes replaying everything – the meds we gave, the arch of his neck with the endotracheal tube in place, the sharp and tangy smell of blood. But I stop myself. Why am I thinking about him *now*? It happened over ten years ago. I don't even know his name. A few years back, I started calling him Daniel. Partly because he looked like a Daniel but mainly because it seemed unfair that he remain nameless after all the years he has crept into my thoughts. I sigh and roll over just as the bedroom door opens. My husband peeks his head inside.

"Dor, it's time to get up."

I groan and check the clock: 10:00 p.m. My attempt at a nap before night shift has proved futile. I rub my eyes. The room is dark, just the way it should be for a restful sleep. Not like during the day when sunlight sneaks through the slats in the blinds. I blink a few times fighting the grogginess.

Bill peels down the covers on his side of the bed. I feel a pang of envy.

"Have you given it any thought? I really think it's time you pack it in. Try your hand at something different. Something with normal hours and weekends off." It's an idea he's been bringing up a lot lately.

I get up and get ready for work. With a quick peck on Bill's cheek I am off, checking on the kids and turning out lights. I lock the door behind me. As I back down the driveway, my headlights illuminate the sleepy house that I wish I was in, tucked beside my husband. I rub my forehead trying to wipe away the dull ache that comes with working nights, and begin reciting my usual prayer: please God, can we keep it light – no emergencies, no palliatives, no heart-wrenching scenarios?

The shift starts out busy: call bells to answer, leftover paperwork from a late evening admission. Plus it's Tuesday, which means it's 'MAR' night, the night we compare our 'medication administration records' with those from the pharmacy. It is a safeguard, another means of ensuring each patient is receiving the drugs that they should be.

Finally, around 3:30 a.m., things begin to settle down. We review our posted schedules, check emails or read updates in the staff notice book. Then a call bell goes off, Room 225. It is Mrs. Glennie, one of my patients, so I get up to answer it. Mrs. Glennie was admitted a few days ago with frequent episodes of shortness of breath, and with a change in medications she's doing much better. In all likelihood she will be discharged in the morning.

As I head down the hallway, I hear a woman moaning. When I get to the room, Mrs. Glennie is rocking back and forth, clutching her right leg.

"Oh nurse, the pain woke me up. It's right here." She points to a specific spot on her calf.

I pull back the covers, my mind automatically recalling an incident years ago when a patient I was caring for developed sudden onset leg pain, just like Mrs. Glennie. On that occasion I wasn't able to palpate a pulse, so I notified the doctor immediately. A Doppler ultrasound confirmed a blood clot large enough to cut off the circulation to the lower leg. Within a half hour, that patient was in surgery. He recuperated without incident. Is that what I am seeing now? I inspect Mrs. Glennie's leg for colour, warmth and sensation. I place my fingers over the area of her pedal pulse and feel nothing. My mind kicks into high gear; since this hospital doesn't have a functioning operating room at night, we will have to transfer her to a facility that does. Time is of the essence. I reposition my hand. Just as I am rechecking for a pulse, Ann, the other RN on duty, comes in. She sizes up the situation. Mrs. Glennie is still moaning and holding her leg. Ann sits Mrs. Glennie up, gently swinging her legs off the side of the bed.

"Okay, let's get you standing. Those leg cramps can be nasty."

A wave of relief spreads over Mrs. Glennie's face. We stand with her at the bedside to ensure the cramp is gone, and I can feel my cheeks flush. When the pain eases off, I help Mrs. Glennie back into bed and Ann returns to the nursing station. Before I pull up Mrs. Glennie's covers I check her legs one more time. The right leg is cool to touch, but so is the left. Not uncommon in a woman of her age and medical condition. Just to be sure, I take the pulse in her foot and behind her knee one more time. Faint but present.

I give my head a shake. How could I have been so off? Why did I immediately assume the worst? And what if I had called the doctor in, only for him or her to discover it was just a charley horse. Thank God, Ann came by.

I give Mrs. Glennie a glass of water, turn off the lights and close the door behind me. Outside the room I take a deep breath. My instinct, that gut feeling I have always relied on, was wrong. It's a skill, fine-tuned and honed over years of experience. Is it something you can lose? I'm not seeing things for what they really are. Jumping to worst-case scenarios. Like everything is a matter of life or death.

And it's not the first time.

A few weeks back, a patient developed chest pain. I was sure he was having a heart attack. Turned out to be indigestion. If I can no longer be objective, it's only a matter of time before my assessments won't be taken seriously. Like the nurse who cried wolf once too often. So far, my judgment has erred on the side of caution, but what happens if in my failure to see things accurately I miss life-threatening symptoms? My stomach knots.

From Mrs. Glennie's room I make my way down the hall to the med room to prepare an intravenous medication that is due shortly. But I can't shake off what just happened. Something's not right. Being on hyper alert for emergency situations is just the half of it. Lately, I've been struggling to get through my shift, to get everything done. It's not workload; all my co-workers seem to be managing. It's the feeling that I can no longer trust myself.

After every shift I drive home worrying about what I might have forgotten. I hate the feeling of getting home and realizing I didn't record a pertinent observation in a patient's chart, or I forgot to check if someone's blood work came back or I didn't call a patient's relative back like they asked. The shift that follows mine is getting used to me phoning once I get home with a list of things I had failed to mention in our change-of-shift reports. The more I obsess over what I might have forgotten to do the more overwhelmed I feel. It's like I'm distracted ... or I just can't seem to prioritize like I used to ... or I'm incompetent. A wave of nausea spreads over me. I don't know what's wrong with me. The only thing I do know is that I'm no longer the nurse I worked so hard to become.

My husband's words come back to me. "Dor, why don't you just quit?" I can't help but wonder if it's time, if a career in nursing has an expiry date and after twenty-two years I've unknowingly exceeded my *best before* date.

Chapter 2

With the boys over at friends for the day, I decide to take my mother out for lunch. She is in town on her annual visit from Calgary and has only three days left before she's due to go home. I suggest the Garden Porch since the day is warm and sunny. With any luck we'll be seated on the patio that overlooks the perennial gardens. Shasta daisies, hostas and day lilies will be in full bloom. My mom loves flowers, and I want to make the most of the time we have left together. She's in her mid-seventies, and lately I can't help thinking, well, that anything can happen at her age. I try not to obsess over it. Awareness of the fragility of life is second nature when you are a nurse.

It's a bit of a drive to the Garden Porch but before long we are south of the city on country roads.

"Mmm, it's beautiful," she sighs, "The sky seems to stretch forever." I look over at her and then follow her gaze to endless fields of wheat, barley and canola. The sky is a pristine blue. Settling back in her seat, she looks so grateful for this moment. I smile and wonder when I last felt like that. Feeling joy in the moment, seeing the world in vivid technicolour, instead of sepia.

"Mom, I think I'm going to hand in my resignation next week."

My mother's eyes widen in surprise. As close as we are, I can't bring myself to admit the real reason for leaving. Not to her or anyone else.

"It will be better for us as a family. We'll be able to get to the cottage every weekend. And I won't have to worry about the boys getting themselves off to school in the morning. Sure they are older now but ..."

Nodding her head she says, "That's good. If you guys can manage it, then that's wonderful." But her look of concern leaves me unconvinced, and my raised eyebrow prompts her to go on.

"No really, I think it's exactly what you need to do. I think it will do you some good." She pauses. "Too much death and sorrow isn't good for anyone." She looks as if she wants to say more, but doesn't.

We decide on the garden vegetable quiche and a spinach salad with clementine oranges and pecans drizzled in blueberry maple dressing. I marvel at the combination of ingredients, things I never would have thought to put together.

"Guess if I do quit, I'll have more time to cook like this. Might even take a couple of cooking courses, you know, like Thai or Indian."

"Or maybe you'll be able to finish that sweater you started knitting last year?"

I laugh, thinking it's more like two years ago. Lengthy projects aren't my thing. Scarves, socks and mittens seem to be the only projects I see through to completion.

Besides, my mother is always sending me hand-knit sweaters. Once again, I am all too aware of how much I will miss her when she's gone. I brush that thought aside, determined to keep our lunch on a light note. We spend the rest of our time discussing things I might do after I "hang up my stethoscope" for good. Putting it like that feels better than to say I'm quitting. Or worse, that I no longer have what it takes.

As we drive home, I feel lighter and more carefree than I have in long time. I want to hang on to that feeling. I want to find joy in random moments like I used to.

*

We are quiet on the drive to the airport. My throat feels thick with words I ought to say, want to say, feel that I can't say. I hate goodbyes. I break the silence, saying that I will try to fly out and visit her and Dad this fall. My mother smiles.

An "oldies" tune comes on the radio. It's been years since I've heard it.

"Hey Mom, remember this song?"

She looks puzzled and stares at the console as if that might tweak her memory.

"It's Babcia's song, remember? Pani Wera's mother?"

Pani Wera and her family were close family friends, so close that we would call her mother Babcia, the polish translation of grandmother. We spent many Sunday afternoons when I was growing up visiting them. They lived on the other side of the city in an area called Little Europe. As we turned onto Euclid Avenue, the aroma of cabbage, pork or beef left simmering on the stove for hours would waft down the street. I knew we were there when we passed the statue of a life-sized angel who stood staring into cupped hands. I always wondered what she was holding.

Babcia lived in the attic. She was old and kept to herself, only coming down to join us for meals. She always wore widow's black, cloaked in sadness. Occasionally, I would ask to visit her and would ascend the long flight of stairs, and then another until I reached the small converted kitchen with its black-and-white tiled floor. And there she would be, sitting in one of the vinyl chairs at her table, her feet crossed and gently swinging, her fingers playing with the starched lace doily, her eyes staring blankly out the window.

I am not sure what attracted me to her. Maybe it was curiosity about death and the toll that grief takes. Maybe it had to do with how secretive it seemed, as if grief itself had taken up residence, and despite attempts to sequester it to the uppermost level, it had an uncanny propensity to seep into the rooms below. Or maybe I was attracted to Babcia's honesty. After all, she was the only one willing to acknowledge the presence of this unwanted tenant.

When mealtime was announced, Babcia was assisted down the stairs to her place at the table filled with steaming hot dishes and usually a creamy sorrel soup. Conversation was light and humorous, except for one occasion. Instead of the usual polkas playing on the record player, a radio played softly in the kitchen. During a brief moment of quiet, the song "Those Were the Days" became more pronounced.

Babcia dropped her soup spoon with a loud clang. She stood, eyes wide with panic, her trembling hands reaching up to cover her ears.

"Mama, I'm sorry, I'll turn it off." Her daughter hurried to the kitchen.

But it was too late. Tears streamed down Babcia's face. She shook her head as if trying to erase the images in her mind that only she could see.

"Come Mama, you should lie down. I'll bring you up some supper later."

When her mother was settled, Pani explained that Babcia could not bear to hear that song. It was a hit years ago, when she was young and newly married. It was one of the many reminders that served to awaken her grief – a song, a picture, the smell of cologne. All too painful to revisit.

There is a lump in my throat and my voice cracks as I refresh my mother's memory of the incident. It's crazy how emotional I can get. I look over at my mother who is watching me with a pained expression, one that says she'd give anything to take away my hurt. I feign a smile and try to laugh off my reaction. She looks away, but I know I haven't fooled her.

Chapter 3

I sit in front of the computer twirling small clumps of hair on the top of my head. I take a strand about the thickness of a pencil and slowly twirl it around my finger. The longer I twist it, the tighter it becomes until eventually it forms a coil that stays put on its own. I move on to the next clump then pat the top of my head. These aren't pretty little ringlets. They look more like corkscrews with tufts of hair sticking out, and they're a bugger to unwind. But it's what I do when I am trying to concentrate.

The computer has switched to screensaver. Little bubbles float down and randomly burst into tiny particles. I've really got to change that, but enough already. I force my hands to the keyboard to write my letter of resignation.

I stare at the screen. So far I have my address in the top right corner with the date below it, and the standard formal greeting. The right words elude me. Maybe it would be easier to write by hand. I reach for a pen, and pause. I keep my pens and pencils in an oversized mug with Nurse written all over it in varying fonts. It was a gift from my mother-in-law. Above it, on the wall, hangs my degree. It took me eight years part time to get that post-diploma Baccalaureate of Science in Nursing. Both boys were born during those years, and were three and five by the time I graduated. I have a picture of them fast asleep, their little bodies draped over the steps leading into the convocation hall, as if sharing the exhaustion of this feat.

I take the mug in my hands curling my fingers around its base. So ... what am I supposed to do with these things? Pack them away? I get a sinking feeling with that thought. I realize that somewhere along the way I have let my career define me, or at least partially, as a person. Wife, mother, nurse. Is wife and mother enough? And what about my Plan B? Every woman needs a Plan B, a means of making it on her own. I've seen far too many widows left poverty stricken. Without my career, where does that leave me?

Bill peers around the door of the office. His eyes widen in surprise and he takes a step back. "Did you know there is a wild animal on your head? Need me to put it out of its misery?"

"Not funny."

"You know, all you need to say is that this is a letter of resignation and that you're giving them two weeks' notice. That's it. Short and simple. Just type that up. Then you can head off to the bathroom to unwind those things."

*

As soon as I arrive at work, I slip the sealed letter into the mail slot for the nursing coordinator. She's in meetings all morning and probably won't see it until early afternoon.

At 2:00 p.m. she finds me in the med room and asks if I have a minute to chat. I've been dreading this all day. We reach her office and she shuts the door, nodding for me to sit in the chair beside her desk.

"I have to tell you this comes as a big surprise."

She picks up my letter and looks directly at me, waiting for me to respond. After much agonizing, I had given no reason for my resignation. I had filled the page with innocuous comments about what a pleasure it had been working with her, the staff and the institution. I don't say anything, and the silence gets awkward.

"So where are you headed?"

The question confuses me at first, and then I realize she thinks I am leaving this job for another.

"Well actually, I'm not going to be nursing at all."

She nods and waits for me to continue. The moment stretches on forever.

"I'm just going to play it by ear for now. Maybe try something new, something completely different."

She's watching me, and I get the sense I am being examined under a microscope. Then she nods, smiles and walks to the door.

"Well, we will certainly miss you."

I get up and follow her out. I let out a heavy sigh, pleased with how well that went. She is obviously used to resignations. Turnover rates in nursing are high. I read a statistic not long ago that thirty to fifty per cent of new nurses consider a change in employment or leave the profession altogether within the first three years of practicing. Although I lasted longer, I suppose I am now another statistic.

Chapter 4

I am dreading this evening, a formal event for my husband's work. I used to love going to these things, but right now I'd much rather put on a comfy pair of PJs and stay in for the night.

As Bill and I mingle with a few people we have never met before, the conversation falls to the topic of occupations. The wife of one of Bill's colleagues, a smartly dressed blonde, goes on at great length about the perks involved with her job as a senior level marketing executive while I stew about what to say. I can't lie and say I am a nurse. I am too young to say I am retired. The few articles I've had published seem hardly enough to call myself a writer. If I say nothing, I'll leave the impression I am a "kept woman," so when it's my turn, I say "I used to be a nurse."

An awkward pause follows, and I feel that everyone in the room can read my guilt at leaving a profession that is experiencing significant shortages. I'm hoping there aren't any other nurses or doctors in the room. A few eyebrows raise, and I brace myself for questions about why I left, knowing I'll sound like a bumbling idiot. I can't explain something I don't fully comprehend myself. But an elderly woman interjects and saves the day.

"Oh, how lovely. You know, I think every family needs a nurse or a doctor. Someone who can help navigate through the health care system that's in place today. Your family is so lucky." She smiles genuinely, and I am grateful to her because the focus is now on the fellow beside me.

*

Bill and I are in the stands of our local hockey arena watching our eldest son's game. Mike started playing hockey when he was six, on defence, but within a couple of years decided he wanted to be a goalie. In my mind there's only one thing worse than being a goalie, and that's being a goalie's mom. Game after game, I watch as he is hammered by slap shots.

It's third period and our team just got a penalty. I sit on the edge of my seat, cringing at the remarks from parents of the opposing team. In no time there's a breakaway. The left winger dekes out our defence, leaving just him and my son. I want to close my eyes but can't. And then it comes. Ten feet from the net, he winds up and takes a shot. The puck hits the top of Mike's helmet and he topples back into the net. I rise to my feet. There is an eerie silence in the arena. It feels like minutes go by but it's really only seconds until Mike gives his head a shake and gets up.

After the game we greet him in the lobby.

"How do you feel?" I begin my questioning. "Does your head hurt? Did you see stars? Did you get dizzy? Do you feel nauseous?"

My husband and son roll their eyes. They have seen me overreact before. Like when Mike had a fever of 39°C and I was sure it was meningitis. Or when Matt, our younger son, had a rash and I spent hours looking on the Internet ruling out everything from Lyme disease to red measles. Even with simple things like splinters, my kids know to go to their dad. When it comes to family, I lose all objectivity. When it comes to family, I get squeamish.

When we get home I ask to see the helmet and immediately notice the small dent from where the puck had hit. I'm not going to take any chances – I will watch him for signs of a concussion. So after Mike gets ready for bed, I explain to him that I will be waking him through the night, just to be sure he is okay.

At 11:00 p.m. I tiptoe into his room. "Mike ... Mike ... can you hear me?"

"Huh?" Mike opens his eyes slowly.

"It's me, does your head hurt?" A few seconds pass. "Mike?" I shake him a little more briskly. "Does your head hurt?"

"No," he says, trying to roll over.

"Wait, I'm just going to have a look in your eyes. Don't mind the bright light." I pull out a pocket flashlight and shine it into his pupils. He squints at the shock of it.

"Mom, I'm fine."

"Okay, okay. But tell me where you are."

"Huh?"

"Where are you right now, this very minute?"

"I'm here, at home. Mom, please let me go back to sleep."

"Okay," I say, "but I'll be back."

I return at 1:00 a.m. and again at 3:00 a.m. Pupils equal and responding briskly to light. Oriented to person, place and time. No headache, no nausea. Irritable, but then maybe that's just because I keep waking him.

At 5:00 a.m., my husband tells me to stay in bed, he'll check on him. I am grateful, but remind him to ask Mike a few key questions. I listen from the warmth of my bed.

"Mike? Mike, can you hear me?"

"Huh? Now you?" Mike is surprised to see his dad.

"Mike, is your mother nuts?"

Mike clears his throat. "Yeah!"

"Okay, nothing wrong with you, go back to sleep."

My husband stumbles back to bed. I decide to forego the 7:00 a.m. check. I lay awake thinking how lucky my family is that I am a nurse.

Chapter 5

For my birthday my husband gives me a three-day kayaking trip. It's something I've always wanted to do but never found the time. Led by a wilderness adventure company called Black Feather, I will be joining a small group of women who will head out in sea kayaks exploring the shores of Georgian Bay. We will be stopping at remote islands, sheltered bays and private beaches to camp each night. As a child, I camped in the area with my parents, and I have never forgotten the beauty of its windswept pines, deep blue waters and rocky outcroppings. All necessary equipment will be provided by the outfitters including food, which will be prepared by our guide. I think I've died and gone to heaven. The trip is advertised as a journey of self-discovery with the opportunity to nurture yourself into feeling whole again. A life coach/Gestalt therapist will accompany us. That part I'm not too sure about.

After a chaotic few days of making sure I am leaving Bill and the boys well stocked with pre-prepared meals, enough clean laundry and an orderly house, I board the plane that will take me to Toronto. From there I've rented a car and will drive to Killbear Provincial Park. I'll stay the night at a local motel and meet up with the group in the morning. This is the first time

I have ever travelled alone, and I am surprised that instead of feeling trepidation I actually love every minute. There is no one complaining about a long flight or a delay in luggage or ...

The motel room is modest and clean, but I inspect the mattress for bedbugs anyway. I rummage through my personal effects double-checking that I have everything on the "What to Bring" list suggested by the outfitters. I can barely contain my excitement and feel like a kid on Christmas Eve. I doubt I'll sleep well tonight. Finally around 11:00 p.m., I lie down on the bed. It's quiet. I look around the room. It's tidy with all of my things in their place. I smile. Why have I never done this before? Take some "me" time.

By noon, our guide has gone over all we need to know about sea kayaks, equipment and our itinerary. Including the guide and the Gestalt therapist, there are eight of us: a mother-daughter pair, two women I suspect are a couple, a university professor and myself. I am paired with Claire, the professor. We'll share a tent at night.

The group sets out onto the water. We're blessed with a warm, sunny day. Our pace is relaxing, there's no hurry to be somewhere by a certain time. As we paddle I watch the shoreline for wildlife or admire the occasional cottage we pass. The water gently laps against the side of my hull. Rock, pine, water. I feel such a sense of peace. The others seem to be feeling it as well because a quiet, reverent mood has taken over. We've all left our troubles behind. It's just the fresh air, this magnificent landscape and us.

We paddle for four or five hours and then find an island that will be perfect for camping. There is even a sandy beach on one side. Setting up tents, collecting wood and building a fire takes a bit of time but before long our guide has something simmering in a pot that smells divine. We feast on a pesto pine nut fusilli served with a salad and fresh bread. Over tea and a berry crumble we get to know each other better. After everyone pitches in to clean up, Lilly, the Gestalt therapist, gathers us together for a little art therapy. She reaches into her knapsack producing paper and trays of watercolour paints. Lilly tells us she believes everyone has an angel looking out for them and asks each of us to think about what our own personal angel would look like.

Finding it hard to concentrate, I sit for a few minutes and then decide to allow myself to play. I apply some paint and watch as it bleeds into the paper. I add more colours, watching how they blend into each other making new colours, varying hues and patterns. Before long, I'm fully immersed in the swirling formations, and when I glance up I notice that the patterns on my page are similar to the wisps of colour in the sky and the rocks surrounding me. And then I begin to see the profile of a face take shape, a well-defined eye and a smile. I am completely lost in this exercise when Lilly tells us it's time to put the paints away. We place our pages on a flat rock to dry.

There is a glorious sunset to watch, and afterwards we stoke the fire and talk long into the night. It is surprising how quickly the group has bonded, sharing parts of ourselves normally restricted to only the closest of friends. To end the perfect day we go for a swim. The still water reflects the moon, and the sky is a burst of stars. I dive in.

The next day is another warm and sunny day. When we stop for lunch, Lilly suggests that she meet with each of us individually to discuss our paintings. Taking my picture from my journal where I stored it for safekeeping, I wait my turn by the water's edge.

"So tell me what you see in your painting." Lilly is sitting cross-legged across from me.

"Well, I see a face." I point out the outline so she can see it as well. "But it's unidentifiable."

"Okay, now I'd like you to turn the page over."

My left eye is watering, and as I turn my page over wondering what I will find, I have to wipe away tears.

"What's wrong with your eye?" Lilly looks mildly concerned.

"Oh, it's nothing, I must have gotten a little sunscreen in it." I motion her to carry on.

"No." Lilly is holding her hand out. "You know, you seem to do that a lot – impose unnecessary discomforts on yourself. This morning when the guide asked if anyone wanted to stop for a bathroom break, you started to raise your hand but when no one else did, you put it back down again, right?"

"Well ... I didn't want to hold everyone up." I think about what Lilly is implying and realize she's right. I often ignore my own needs. And actually, for no good reason at all. I get up and rinse water on my face. The stinging in my eye ceases immediately.

Seeing my relief, Lilly says, "Remember that," accentuating every syllable. "Martyrdom sucks." I smile sheepishly at her like I've just been scolded for not knowing a fundamental truth.

We spend another amazing afternoon on the water and by dinner we are all famished. Our guide prepares yet another succulent meal: a shrimp stir fry with rice and fresh vegetables. The meal comes complete with a fortune cookie. I eat my cookie first then unfold the small white paper and read it aloud. *If you make yourself a mouse, you raise the possibility of being eaten by a cat.* I decide to try another one, hoping for a little more upbeat fortune, but when I open the paper it is exactly the same. We all laugh.

"No escaping the truth." Lilly looks over at me with a smug smile.

By the end of our trip I am reluctant to say goodbye to my new friends. I have grown very close to two of the women, and we promise to try to keep in touch. As I drive away toward the highway, I get the sense that I just experienced something "otherworldly." Like I was plucked out of everyday life and placed on a surreal journey to bliss.

On the plane ride home I settle into my seat, placing my book in the seat pocket along with headphones and my iPod. The airline attendant begins the usual safety spiel: "In the event of an emergency, oxygen masks will be released. Be sure to secure one on yourself before assisting others ..." How many times I have flown and never really heard the meaning behind those words? Take care of yourself first. Don't make yourself a mouse. It's not selfish, it's responsible. If you don't help yourself first, you'll never be able to help anyone else.

Chapter 6

"No!" A muffled scream escapes from my throat and jolts me awake. I sit up, heart racing. I look around and realize that I am at home, in bed. It was only a dream. I take a deep breath, trying to calm my nerves as images come back to me.

I was at work trying to get to a patient in critical condition, but things kept happening to stop me. A patient pushing an IV pole stumbled and fell to the floor in a crumpled heap, the pole smashing down on top of him. A woman restrained in a geriatric chair was trying to pry her way loose shouting, "Nurse, nurse, help me."

Everywhere I looked IV bags had run dry and blood was backing up in the tubing. Call bells were going off. I was trying to get the morning medications out but was so far behind that doses would be missed altogether. Abandoning the medication cart, I headed to the patient's room and as I entered, the alarm from his cardiac monitor went off. I looked up at the screen and saw the rapid, irregular arching waves of ventricular fibrillation, a lethal arrhythmia. I ran to the bedside. His skin was already ashen grey, his eyes rolled back as the life drained out of him. That's when I woke up.

I glance at the blue glare of the clock radio: 3:17 a.m. Every muscle in my body is tense. I take a few deep breaths and try to relax. Just another one of those "over the top" dreams where the mouse of my daytime worries has a way of turning into an elephant at night. Or at least what used to be my daytime worries. It's been well over a year since I left nursing. Bill is asleep bedside me, his breathing slow and rhythmic. I squeeze my eyes shut hoping to hang on to any thread of drowsiness, but it's too late, sleep has eluded me again.

I get up, grab a sweater and tiptoe from our bedroom, winding my way around spots on the floor that I know will creak. It's a path that's become all too familiar. Veer to the left by the boys' bedroom, a bit to the right by the bathroom, skip the first stair going down. A bluish hue of light from the microwave illuminates the last few steps to the kitchen where I fill the kettle with water for a cup of camomile tea.

Why am I still plagued by these dreams? It seems absurd, as if part of me just can't let go. The details of the dreams change, but the theme is usually the same: I can't seem to get done what needs to be done.

And then there are those memories that play back at random times. Like the other day at the grocery store. I picked up a package of ground beef without realizing the cellophane had a tear in it, and a drop of blood trickled out and fell to the floor. Staring at it, I was instantly back at the bedside caring for a patient with a bleeding ulcer, holding a basin under his chin as he vomited, splatters of bright red blood landing on his gown, the sheets and the tiled floor. Between the crazy dreams at night and the obtrusive thoughts in the day, I'm beginning to feel haunted by all that I've seen and done in my years as a nurse. I wonder if I'm losing my mind.

I take the mug of tea to my office where stacks of reading material provide refuge from late night thoughts. I turn the computer on, my eyes drawn to the colour of the "on" button. My home is filled with neon blue lights at night.

I click on Google and type in "burnout," one of the most commonly cited reasons for people leaving careers in health care. The term has been around for years and is generally understood to mean a lack of satisfaction with a job as a result of feeling overworked, overstressed and undervalued. Burnout can leave you feeling exhausted, dissatisfied and depressed. Check, check and check. But reading through the list of symptoms, I feel a familiar irritation growing in the pit of my stomach. I've read that same list dozens of times and each time I react the same way – defensively. That's not it. There's more to it. I may have had some burnout, but that's not why I left.

Frustrated, I exit from that website and am redirected to the CNN homepage showing live coverage of a fatal shooting at a small town factory: three people killed, gunman shot by police, workers to get trauma counselling. The last line surprises me, and yet it shouldn't. Natural disasters, acts of violence, rape and abuse can happen to anyone, and any of those can result in post-traumatic stress disorder (PTSD). It is not just soldiers of war who suffer from trauma. Imagine going to work expecting the usual routine only to have everything thrown into chaos by the unmistakeable sound of gunshots? The fear they must have felt.

I type in post-traumatic stress disorder and hit search. It comes back with three million hits. Well, that ought to make me sleepy. At least I'm not thinking about my own troubles anymore.

The first few sites review the history of PTSD. I read about soldiers in World War I diagnosed with hysteria, mental collapse or cowardice in a time when little was known or understood about the condition. Labelled "malingerers," they were considered weak and unmanly, often shamed into returning to the frontlines. On one page there's a photograph with the caption "Soldier's Heart – WWI." It must have been taken after one of those horrific battles like Ypres, Somme or Passchendaele. Carnage is everywhere. Charred stumps are all that remain of trees. Buildings are reduced to rubble. Off to one side a young soldier sits slumped against a rock, his uniform bloodied and torn, his bayonet tossed carelessly aside. He is glassy eyed, as if he's not all there. His expression haunts me. I can't begin to imagine the horrors he's witnessed. I can't imagine having to plunge a bayonet into another human being, even if he is an enemy. I inhale deeply and look at the soldier again. The nerve endings on the back of my neck tingle. There is something familiar about him. I wonder if we could be related. No, my family comes from Europe and weren't even in Canada during the Great War.

My attention is drawn to my Nurse mug. I take another deep breath. "Something's not right with me." My words come out in a whisper. "As long as I keep pretending everything is okay, it never will be." Saying the words out loud feels right; I am finally admitting something. I think about the dreams and disturbing memories. How I can no longer face sickness or sorrow without feeling like I'll fall apart.

I print off the page with the photograph of the soldier and pin it to the bulletin board. I turn off the computer and head back to bed.

As I crawl under the covers, the image of the soldier stays with me. Bill is still asleep, undisturbed by my night-time ritual. We are so different, the two of us. When he is troubled by something, he sleeps. It completely baffles me how, but I've seen it so often over the years that I no longer question it. And right now, I envy it. I close my eyes and allow the rhythm of his breathing to relax me. I try to match the sequence as if we are dancing. With every inhalation we take a step to the right, with every exhalation we sweep to the left.

Finally, sleep overcomes me.

Chapter 7

Between raising our sons, the busy years of either building or renovating homes and juggling Bill's work schedule with my career, I can't help but feel that my husband and I are drifting apart. The last time we went to a movie together was eight years ago, to see *Titanic*. I can't remember our last romantic dinner. But it is not just life circumstances that have gotten in our way. I have changed.

As I am folding laundry, Bill comes up behind me and encircles me in his arms. In the last few years we have become less and less demonstrative, so this small gesture feels almost intrusive. Instead of a show of affection, it feels like an infringement of space. I step from his embrace and ask about the boys' hockey schedule. If Bill takes offense by my actions, he doesn't let on.

Later, when I am in bed reading, I hear him switching off all the lights. He goes into the bathroom to brush his teeth and undress. A familiar trepidation comes over me. I turn out the lamp on my side of the bed and feign sleep. When he climbs into bed, he rests his arm on mine. It's one of those unspoken cues between couples that signify wants, desires, intentions. I don't move. His hand begins sliding gently from my shoulder to my elbow. I squeeze my eyes shut trying to convince myself that we ought to, it's been weeks. Bill has been so patient with all of my excuses, no matter how lame. I try and muster up whatever I need to, but simply can't.

"Oh gosh, I completely forgot to send an email." I hop out of bed and put on a housecoat. Bill sighs and rolls over.

I stumble into my office and plunk myself down in my chair. Relief spreads over me. I'll wait a few minutes; surely he'll be asleep when I go back in. I shake my head, hardly believing what's become of us, or more correctly, me. It's not the physical I shy away from, it's the emotional. And it's not just with Bill. I have slowly distanced myself from many old and dear friends as well.

The photo of the soldier catches my eye and I unpin the picture to examine it. Once again the hairs on my neck stand on edge. His expression is what gets me each time I look at him. He is broken. I stare awhile longer and begin to realize why he seems familiar. Because in him, I see me.

I lean back in my chair and think about what it must have been like for the men who enlisted, many as young as eighteen. The rat and lice-infested trenches lined with sandbags to keep the sides from collapsing, the deafening sound of intense artillery bombardment, the pungent, metallic smell of blood mixed with gunpowder. I imagine injured soldiers being taken to first aid posts and then transferred to base hospitals as required. It must have been a relief to find yourself in one of the many cots that lined the white-washed walls of makeshift hospital wards, away from the steady barrage of gunfire. No doubt nightfall would transform the ward into chaos, as horrors replayed themselves and men awakened screaming, a few requiring several people to restrain them. The ghosts have returned.

As physical injuries healed, men were told to *suck it up, take it like a soldier. Get back to the front.* They were told there was no room for emotion in a soldier's life. They were accused of being weak in character. Doctors, pressured by the brass ranks to get any able-bodied men back to the front, knew they were sending the lamb to the lion. Many returned to the front, their non-physical symptoms worse. A few chose desertion. When they were caught, they were tried and shot. Some men were mute, others had limbs that shook violently, and many had glazed, empty expressions. It caused a stir in the medical community. What was this ailment? At first they believed it was a result of an explosion to the brain. They sent the worst of the men to psychiatric facilities all over England where they received the latest treatment known as Faradism, which involved the application of electrical currents to various parts of the body. Mute soldiers had the stimulus applied to the back of their throats. The lame had it applied to their back and legs. Some endured treatment for hours on end, to no avail.

A few innovative doctors began to believe this state was caused by the horror of what these men had witnessed, horrors that had become trapped in a circuit-like pattern of thought. They advised rest and relaxation as well as therapy to unlock the thought process.

I look at the photo of the soldier. Maybe he was diagnosed with "shell shock," the term used during World War I. The terminology changed in World War II to "combat neurosis" and "battle fatigue." It wasn't until the Vietnam War that post-traumatic stress was recognized. Prior to that, soldiers not only suffered the symptoms of PTSD, but the wrath of the military and lack of treatment from a health care system that didn't understand what they were dealing with.

I return to my own battle: how I ended up feeling incapable of doing my job, how I avoid facing situations that remind me of sickness or death. The nightmares and intrusive thoughts. The loss of joy, the panic that rises to the surface with little provocation. Even though I have never been to war, my symptoms are so similar to those of PTSD that it seems like a logical starting point. I read through several articles. One is about animal care workers who suffer from trauma while caring for abused and beaten animals. They refer to it not as PTSD but secondary traumatic stress (STS). I read the definition: its symptoms and the words start humming.

Secondary traumatic stress, also known as compassion fatigue, is defined as the natural behaviours and emotions that result from helping or wanting to help a traumatized or suffering person.[1] It is considered *the cost of caring*. Healers, helpers or rescuers are all at risk. It can also be an occupational hazard for lawyers, journalists, veterinarians, teachers – anyone who assists those who have suffered trauma. The concept first surfaced in the mid- to late 1980s. Since then, thanks to pioneers in the field of traumatology like Dr. Charles Figley, knowledge of STS has grown exponentially.

Although no one is immune, not all health care personnel experience symptoms of STS. Further studies into the reasons behind this and ways to decrease susceptibility are needed.

Secondary traumatic stress is often confused with burnout, a concept introduced in the mid-1970s to describe a state of frustration, powerlessness and inability to achieve work goals.[2] Although some symptoms are similar to STS – for example, emotional exhaustion and depersonalization (when you feel hardened by the job) – the diagnoses are not the same. In general, burnout focuses on the work environment, the workload and job satisfaction. Burnout, like STS, can have a gradual onset and worsen over time. But unlike STS, symptoms can often be alleviated by time off, or a change in work environment or work assignment. Over the years, burnout has become the "go to" term for people believing the stress of their jobs is getting to them. But assuming burnout may mean missing the signs of STS, which can have far more debilitating symptoms.

The onset of STS can occur on any given day while witnessing the suffering of others – a single defining moment that alters everything. With repeated exposure to the suffering of others, symptoms progress until the condition is almost indistinguishable from PTSD. Although each person will experience STS differently, key symptoms such as recurring thoughts and dreams, altered perception and judgment, and a sense of helplessness set in. Without intervention, life as you know it can change. A loss of joy, withdrawal from intimacy, episodes of depression, and even suicide, are all possible.

Even though the symptoms are all negative, relief spreads over me as I realize I am finally onto something. My thoughts automatically go to nursing, to all the hurt and heartache I've witnessed – memories that stay with me like a wound that won't heal. It has been over a year since I left and the wound is now bleeding into my personal life. Avoidance has become my bandage, which is fine for little cuts and scrapes, but when you cover up an infected wound, it will fester.

Several hours later I look up from the computer screen. A pinkish orange glow is transforming the night sky. Stars fade against the brilliance of the rising sun and its promise of a new day. I stretch, my back aching from spending the night in my chair. On my desk is a list. *Ways I Have Changed*. I've written a long list of items, starring the ones that impact my personal life. *Distancing myself* and *loss of hope* have double stars. Those are the symptoms that bother me most, that have changed me the most.

I look again at the soldier. I feel inexplicably grateful to him, as if he knows what I am feeling and is prompting me on.

I decide that in order to get to the bottom of all this, I will need to peel back the gauze covering my wounds. I will need to venture into the memories I have carefully locked away and labelled *Admittance Prohibited*. I owe it to my family, my friends. I owe it to myself.

If I head to bed now, I'll get a couple of hours of sleep before the boys get up. I take the photo of the soldier and clip the picture to a fresh page. At the top of the page I write *What Happened?*

Part Two
1979–2005

All the art of living lies in a fine mingling
of letting go and holding on.
—Haveback Ellis

Chapter 8

I hold my breath to steady my hand. With a quick flick of my wrist I plunge the needle deep into the dimpled skin of an orange. I've been told it's good to practice on an orange; its texture is similar to skin. And so I do. I don't want to be one of those nurses who give needles that hurt. I imagine my patients saying, "I hardly even felt that" or "Wow, that didn't hurt a bit!" But as I examine the remaining length of needle sticking out of my orange, I know if I had been giving that injection to a real patient, it would have hit bone. Ouch.

Start all over again: landmark the site; swab with alcohol; say, "Okay, you'll feel a poke."

I go through each step, getting a feel for the depth and angle of penetration. How many oranges have I gone through? Bushels? It doesn't matter because when it comes time for testing, we will be giving saline-filled injections to our lab partners ... and I happen to like mine. I reach for another orange.

Denise and I became lab partners on our first day of class. We are both the same age and just out of high school.

"Find yourselves a partner. Don't worry about whether you know each other; you'll become very acquainted during the course of the semester."

I don't know anyone, and neither does Denise. Since we both stand there looking awkward, we gravitate toward each other, oblivious to what the role of lab partner really means. Within a short time we have it figured out: we are each other's guinea pigs. We will practice many different skills on each other before we try them out on real patients.

I love the lab. When I enter through the large swinging doors, the smell of disinfectant and freshly laundered sheets greets me. Hospital beds are lined up along the wall, and a wide variety of equipment like blood pressure cuffs and stethoscopes, IV poles and k-basins are ready for use. It is a simulated hospital environment. There are mannequins, some full bodied, others just body parts such as an arm with thick ropey veins waiting for an IV, or a perineum dreading the probe of a catheter. The lab is where we put theory into practice, the place where we go to become fully immersed in the world of nursing.

We start out in the lab learning the basics such as taking blood pressure, temperature and pulse. Over the months, the skills we learn increase in complexity: dressing changes for a variety of wounds, delivering injections and managing intravenous drips. Stethoscopes fascinate me. I adjust the earpieces so that they are angled slightly forward and pay particular attention to the resonance. I listen carefully to the sounds of air as it enters and exits the lungs. I imagine the exchange of gases, oxygen in, and carbon dioxide out. I move on to the whooshing noise of the heart and listen to the valves clamping shut within the chambers. It is exciting to experience the body through sound.

It is chilly in the lab, the temperature probably lowered on purpose to drive home what it feels like to be chilled and exposed as a patient. Our professor walks around, pointing out things we're doing wrong.

"And don't let me see you wearing gloves when you are just taking blood pressure. Can you imagine how impersonal that would feel?"

We quickly learn that awareness of the patient's feelings is paramount in nursing – everything from explaining procedures in detail before they are performed in the hopes of alleviating fear, to understanding how hospitals can leave people feeling so vulnerable.

The lab is my haven, a safe place to try out new skills and practice them over and over. There is great comfort in knowing that if something doesn't go just right, you simply try again. But the inevitable is pending: our first clinical rotation is drawing near, and the pretend world of nursing will soon be replaced with the real McCoy.

When the day finally arrives, my father offers to drive me to the hospital since it's close to where he works. I hurry him out to the car. I want to get there early. We drive in silence. He occasionally looks over at me with what seems like a sense of pride, and this surprises me because he did his best to discourage me from going into nursing. "Why would you want to be a nurse, when you could be a doctor?"

My palms are sweaty, I have a dull ache in my forehead and I can't stop chewing on the inside of my cheek. I fight to keep my breakfast down. Uniform, shoes, cap, pocket protector with pen, pencil and flashlight. On the radio, "Mellow Yellow" is playing. I look out the car window and watch the city come to life in the early morning hour: people waiting at bus stops, office lights flickering on, a dog scrounging for scraps. Somehow I will have to fit into this new life I have chosen for myself. Somehow I will have to leave the security of the lab behind.

§§§

In nursing school, we are taught to consider patients' feelings first. Numerous studies concur that when patients receive compassionate care, they experience more positive outcomes such as increased satisfaction and a willingness to follow through with their treatment.[3] But it is not just the patient who benefits. As compassion develops, the rapport between patient and care provider moves to another level. The desire to help increases and accentuates the sense of satisfaction we gain. We feel good about ourselves.

Human beings are wired in such a way that we become emotionally entangled; a caring look or smile becomes a current of comfort flowing from one person to another, whereas the high voltage of any negative emotions can electrocute. Beneath the threshold of conscious awareness, our sensitive antennae pick up on the signals others are sending. When someone stubs his toe, we wince. When we hear a child crying, our heart goes out to them. When we see a widow grieving, we feel sad.

The root of compassion takes hold early in life. Studies have shown that children as young as two years old have the ability to feel distress toward another being.[4] Our childhood experiences shape our abilities to reach out to others in compassionate ways. Upbringing often sets the stage for this, and the capacity to respond to one another continues to develop.

In training, we are taught to empathize, not sympathize. To sympathize suggests pity, which has a way of making a person a victim. Empathy is the ability to understand what someone else is feeling. It is like stepping into another person's shoes in order to grasp what they are going through. It is the prerequisite emotion for developing compassion. And it is at the heart of STS.

Each of us sees the world through different filters. Some hearts are more responsive than others. In her book *The Highly Sensitive Person*, Elaine Aron describes a trait (not a disorder) found in approximately fifteen to twenty per cent of the population. This innate trait has characteristics such as the ability to take in subtleties that others miss, an intuitive nature, and the tendency toward increased emotional responsiveness. She claims that while twenty per cent are extremely sensitive, another twenty-two per cent are moderately sensitive.[5] If highly sensitive people choose careers in health care, could this increase the risk of developing STS? It would seem logical. The old axiom "healer know thyself" rings true when it comes to compassion. Knowing your own degree of responsiveness to the suffering of others can be critical in understanding how to prepare yourself for a career in any of the caring professions, not to mention life in general. Knowing how to separate yourself from all that you see, yet still be engaged enough to fully understand, is a delicate balance.

Chapter 9

I enter the hospital through its front revolving doors. As I push on the handle it seems to scoop me up and toss me inside like a reluctant child caught dawdling. A group of fellow student nurses gathers in the lobby. The instructor arrives and steers us toward the elevators, down to the basement and to the locker rooms. We change in silence, donning crisp white uniforms, carefully pinning our caps in place with bobby pins. I steal a glance at myself in a full-length mirror and a nasty voice in my head says, "Who are you kidding?"

I am paired with Suzanne, an RN who is not much older than me. She takes me aside to go over how I can help and places a hand on mine. "Hey, relax. I promise – no brain surgery today." I flush at the thought of being so transparent. I spend the day taking blood pressures and pulses, making beds and giving bed baths. I watch Suzanne carefully: the way she assesses her patients, how she interacts with them, how she organizes her time. She is an excellent role model. I go home tired but relieved.

By the end of the first year I have adjusted to the pace, juggling clinical rotations with time spent in class or in the lab learning new skills, and the endless hours of study. We have gone from being at the hospital once a week to three days a week.

"Make sure you come prepared."

The instructor's tone leaves no room for misunderstanding. Each day we are quizzed about our patients. How are they progressing, why are they on certain meds, how does their illness affect their life? The difficulty of questions steadily increases.

I spend most weekends with my head in the books reading about diseases, their symptoms and treatments. I study various medications and their side effects until I can recite them in my sleep. Anatomy and physiology become increasingly complex: glomerular filtration in the nephrons of the kidney, how Kupffer cells and hepatocytes function, the release of vasopressin in response to plasma osmolarity, blood pressure and blood volume. Every organ and body system is stripped down to its cellular level. I read up on my assigned patients' previous history. It dawns on me that I know my patients' medical histories better than I know my own relatives'.

Occasionally a few of us get together for drinks, where inevitably the conversation drifts to plans after graduation. Denise and I want to go to California, but we try not to get too far ahead of ourselves. Classmates around us are dropping out or failing at an alarming rate. And we don't want to be one of them. By the completion our program, we will have lost almost half of our classmates.

*

My first experience with death occurs during my first semester of training. We are assigned to a med/surgical unit, and at the start of the shift our clinical instructor gathers us together to inform us of a death on the unit. "It will be a good opportunity to go over the care of a deceased body," she says as we are ushered into the room.

The only time I've ever seen a dead body was when I was around ten, at the funeral of a distant relative. I can't even say I saw the body; all I really remember is peeking around the arms of my father who was doing his best to shield me from seeing.

I enter the room with trepidation, accosted by the staleness of the air. The man had been sick for a long time. Lying on the bed, covered in a white sheet, is a lifeless body. As our instructor folds back the sheet, I am struck by the man's frozen expression of awe. His eyes focus intently on the ceiling. His jaw hangs loose in amazement. What did he see in those last few moments of life? The instructor proceeds to talk about the care of a body, gently closing his eyelids and replacing his dentures. She tells us it is important to get the dentures in before rigor mortis sets in, otherwise it will be too difficult. Each of us is encouraged to touch the body. I place my hand on his arm, surprised by the warmth that still remains. By the mottling that is already occurring on the undersides of his body, I know that this warmth is draining out with each passing moment.

The room is still, each of us thinking our own thoughts. One student nurse wipes tears from her eyes, and I learn later that she lost her father a few years ago. I am surprised by my own reaction, or lack of it. I can't say I feel sad. Respect and reverence, yes, but somehow I feel removed from emotion. Instead, I concentrate on what I need to know about the care of a deceased body. I take in every detail, remove any catheters or IVs, and take note of where to apply the labels of identification and how to wrap the body in the body bag. For now I am totally focused on what I need to know.

§ § §

In 2006, a study was undertaken to determine if levels of empathy of medical students changed at all during their training. Students at the Boston University School of Medicine were surveyed in all four years utilizing The Jefferson Scale of Physician Empathy – Student version. The surprising results were published in 2007 in the *Journal of General Internal Medicine*.[6] Chen et al. found that empathy levels gradually decreased over the four years. Naturally, this prompted a critical look at how physicians were being trained.

When I compared this disturbing finding with my own experience, it only served to raise more questions about the intricate workings of empathy and compassion. If we are cognitively engaged in completing a procedure or learning something new, is it possible that those activated regions of the brain take precedence over the limbic or emotional portions? Can both parts of the brain fire intensely at the same time? Is there a dimmer switch for emotional thinking? Is opening up to feel compassion something we do consciously or subconsciously? And if we do so consciously, is it something we can turn on or off? If, when we open ourselves and it becomes too painful, can we switch gears somehow so as not to become overwhelmed?

With so many questions yet to be answered, it is a promising sign that research on compassion has grown considerably in the last two decades. Functional MRI scans have enabled scientists to map various regions in the brain associated with compassion. Experts recognize that it is not just in the mind that we experience compassion; our bodies are tuned in as well. Neuropeptides and neurohormones, found not only in the brain but also in various parts of the body such as the heart, the lining of the gut and lungs, are released in response to emotions. These neurochemicals change the state of cells within the body. When we engage in compassionate behaviour, for example, oxytocin floods our brains eliciting a "feel good" response.

For many years, researchers could not agree on a definition for compassion. Today, many experts concur that compassion is a multidimensional process that includes (a) a cognitive function of being aware of the suffering, (b) an affective component that includes being emotionally moved by the suffering, (c) an intention or wish to see the suffering relieved, and (d) a motivational component that becomes the action taken to help relieve the suffering.[7]

His Holiness the Dalai Lama has said, "The cultivation of compassion is no longer a luxury but a necessity if our species is to survive." Being compassionate toward one another has a significant impact on the greater good; it is at the core of humanity and is said to positively affect pleasure, immunity and well-being.

But being compassionate can pose risks. The key to providing compassionate care is understanding the delicate balance at play. Too much and you'll be burned, too little and the care isn't as effective.

At this point in my training, however, I was so immersed in learning that I gave little thought to the inner workings of compassion. Concentrating on the skills of patient care, I headed blindly into my career.

Chapter 10

On convocation day, I stand in my black flowing robe amid fellow nursing students clasping my diploma as we recite a modified version of the Nightingale Pledge, the nursing version of the Hippocratic Oath, promising to practice our profession faithfully, to maintain confidentiality and to devote ourselves to the welfare of those committed to our care. When the ceremony comes to an end, I join the others in tossing my cap high into the sky. As the black discs come tumbling down, a nagging suspicion surfaces in my mind. Am I ready?

Dreams of moving to California had fizzled out during our final year when nursing jobs in Ontario went from being scarce to abundant almost overnight. I am hired on a med/surgical unit at one of the Toronto hospitals where I did much of my clinical training. Miss Cooper, the head nurse, often comes in on her days off. She rules her ward like a military unit, complete with thorough inspections of each nurse's appearance as we arrive for our shifts. No nail polish, no loose strands of hair, and absolutely no jewellery. Once approved, the day can begin. It is the last few years of white uniforms, starched crisp.

The first few years are trying. Filled with uncertainties, unknowns and some of the biggest fears I have ever faced. But none as riveting as the loss of life itself.

*

Jim has bone cancer. Recently remarried, and obviously in love, both he and his wife are clinging to a glimmer of hope that the endless rounds of chemotherapy might allow him more time. When he arrived on our unit, the cancer had spread extensively involving his spine, pelvis and long bones. Pain is something he lives with daily.

I like Jim. I admire the brave face he puts on, his quick wit and easy-going manner and the way no gesture, however small, goes unnoticed. As the weeks pass, we grow closer. He comes as a package, complete with dedicated wife and two courageous kids. I get to know them almost equally as well and can't help but worry about how they are coping. Rooted in the reality of his lab tests and x-rays, I keep things light, sensing that's what he needs right now – and not wanting to burst the bubble of hope he is clinging to. But I don't want to instill any false hope either. I can't help but wonder what will happen when his façade comes crumbling down. With each passing day, my concern intensifies.

At the start of one evening shift, I enter Jim's room and find him alone. His most recent CAT scan results had come back, and the doctor was in earlier to inform him. The cancer has spread to his lungs. He is struggling to reposition himself in bed but the effort is too much. He is in a lot of pain. Beads of sweat form on his forehead and his skin is ashen grey. When he notices me, his grimace turns into a smile. I am beginning to see a pattern developing; he is in the habit of declining his pain meds each afternoon, withholding them until after his family leaves.

"So, any news yet? Did Kevin make the team?" Jim's son made it to the final cut of his school baseball team.

"Don't know yet, he should be here soon." He arches his back to alleviate some of the discomfort.

"How about I get you something for your pain?"

"No thanks, I don't want them to see me all doped up."

I understand his dilemma. He is torn between being in the moment with a great deal of pain, or vaguely remembering the visit with his kids.

"But you're okay with them seeing you like this?" He looks at me and shrugs as if to pass it off.

"Okay, but let's get you turned and freshened up." I lift his arm gently; his bones are fragile as toothpicks and he already has a fractured tibia. He hollers out in pain. I stop and let him catch his breath. I take a much-needed breath, too.

"Jim, please let me bring you something." Am I pleading with him because I can't stand to see him in such pain?

Tears steam down his face and he begins to sob. I pull up a chair and sit down, placing a hand over his. We sit like this for a few moments before he can speak.

"There is still so much I have to say to them."

I listen as Jim shares some of his biggest fears: Will they be okay? How will all this affect them? Will they remember him? His pent up thoughts spew forth like lava from a volcano. So much unfinished business, so much he still needs to do. He decides that he must talk to them today. His words are raw and filled with pain. I am uncomfortable and wish I were more experienced so that I might offer words of comfort, but I have nothing to give except my presence.

Jim is finishing off when his family arrives. Both Jim and I have red, puffy eyes. Our appearance gives them the heads up. In the moments to follow, they too will look like us. Jim will speak to his family and do his best to tell them all that he has left to say.

It was one of the last few days Jim stoically managed his pain. For the remainder of his short, well-lived life, he is heavily medicated. With his wife at his bedside, he opens his eyes and greets me, a wash of relief spreading across his face. We exchange smiles, and he drifts off to sleep.

After a few days off, I return to work and go directly to Jim's room. I enter cautiously, knowing what I might find. An empty bed. Choking back tears, I hear footsteps behind me. It is Miss Cooper. She places her arm around my shoulders, revealing her softer side.

"Jim died a peaceful death on Saturday, his wife and kids were here. I know the two of you were close. I wish I could say it gets easier, but really ... it doesn't."

After work I take a walk in hopes of clearing my mind. But I can't stop thinking, why him? Why, at a point in his life when he had so much to hope and live for? Why?

I eventually find myself at the edge of a pond. I spot something on a reed and stoop to look more closely. It is a dragonfly naiad. I watch as it struggles to emerge from its shell, first its upper torso, then its lower until it finally breaks free. It takes a few gulps of air as it waits for its body to expand and for the blood to flow into its wings. This is when it is most vulnerable. Like the naiad, I am adjusting to a new identity. What I don't realize is how vulnerable I am. With that similarity lost on me, I take a few deep breaths and head for home.

§§§

As naïve as it may be, when I first decided to become a nurse, I never gave much thought to how much exposure to death and dying I would have. I envisioned myself helping people get better, easing their pain and improving their quality of life. I had given no thought to what it would be like to lose a patient or having to speak to the family when I did. The loss of a life felt like failure.

In hindsight, I could have made it easier on myself by not attaching an outcome to the care I provided. Asking "why" is futile; we will never have the answers in this lifetime. Focusing on providing the best possible care is all you can do.

No one ever really knows what will happen. The young man with pneumonia isn't supposed to die. The frail elderly man's chances of recovery are slim, but he beats the odds. You can only focus on the here and now, and leave what will be to the powers that be.

Throughout my career, I always felt as if the grief I experienced when losing certain patients was not really mine to feel. But I was wrong. When you care for people, regardless of whether you have known them for a few hours, days or years, you develop a rapport with them. You need to give yourself permission to work through the emotions it stirs up. I shouldn't have attempted to bury my emotions or dismiss them as unimportant. Unresolved grief is toxic.

Rituals have always been widely used in grief healing, and it may have been helpful for me to establish a ceremonial act such as writing a letter to the deceased and burning it afterwards, planting a seed in the person's honour or throwing stones into a river and with each toss imagining the sadness being unleashed. It is far worse to bottle those emotions.

Chapter 11

With a few years of med-surgical experience under my belt, I begin to feel more at ease. Responsibilities like assuming the role of nurse in charge come easier as I learn to trust in myself. Each time I face a difficult situation, my confidence level grows. On several occasions, I witness the code blue team in action, and watch in fascination how the nurses on the team conduct themselves. They are knowledgeable and confident in their skills as they hook up equipment, start IVs and administer life-saving drugs. Their added training allows them to perform advanced procedures and give certain medications without the presence of a doctor. To me, they seem a calibre above the rest of us, and I want to become one of them.

I begin the additional studies required. I take night school classes and use vacation time to take intensive week-long courses. Learning to read an electrocardiogram is like learning a new and exotic language. For months, I stare at the wavelike formations on the page wondering if they will ever make sense. Determined not to give up, I take more courses. And finally one day, like a fog has been lifted, the waves, the spikes, the shapes begin to have meaning. Not long after, I am hired in the Coronary Care Unit (CCU).

Specializing in coronary care proves to be a good fit for me. The defined focus allows me to feel more in control and self-assured. Before long I am hooked on the fast-paced, high-intensity nature of the job. I love the adrenalin rush of emergency situations, the sense of accomplishment in snatching patients back from the grip of death, and knowing we did all we could for those we couldn't save. I feel that I've finally found my niche.

One of the roles of a CCU nurse is to carry the "code blue" pager. In the event of a cardiac arrest anywhere in the hospital, the CCU nurse is part of the team of responders who have advanced training in resuscitation. Each shift, one nurse is assigned to carry the pager. Tonight that nurse is me.

Shortly after 11:00 p.m., the pager goes off. Trauma Room 3 in Emergency. When I arrive the room is empty except for the emergency room doctor.

"Three car pile-up on the 401, first ambulance just arrived, four victims in total, looks like we are in for a busy night."

He is flatline when they bring him in. CPR in progress as the stretcher enters the trauma room. I catch a glimpse of him: a young man, a large flap of his scalp held in place by blood-stained gauze.

"Seventeen-year-old male in an MVA. Right front passenger, belted, car broadsided from the right. Vital signs absent."

Immediately, we go to work. I begin drawing up medications while the emergency room nurse starts an intravenous and administers the sodium bicarb. The physician inserts an endotracheal tube.

"Epinephrine 5mL." I glance at the clock to record the time I administer it.

"Can you take over bagging?" The doctor hands me the resuscitator bag. I attach it to oxygen tubing, give it a few good squeezes, then begin to rhythmically compress the bag in sequence with the compressions.

"Anything yet?"

We all stop briefly and watch the monitor. It is unchanged. Asystole. Flatline.

"Nothing, keep up with compressions."

We continue our efforts. I wipe the blood from this young man's face, a nice-looking kid. What a shame, someone so young. I wonder if anyone is with him. From where I am standing I can see another patient in the adjacent treatment room, a woman who appears to be in her forties, with the same jet-black hair and similar facial features. Most likely his mother. There is a flurry of activity surrounding her. I see her straining to see into this room. Her eyes move from her son, to me and back to him. A wave of torment spreads across her face. A desperate moan escapes from her, and she reaches her hand out to him. Then she looks at me pleadingly. Before I know what is happening I am caught up in the moment as though a vibrational force swirls around this woman, her son and me. Time seems suspended. I am struck with her anguish; everything else fades into the background. A lump forms in my throat. It is as if a window into her emotions has opened and I am seeing things as she is. Even though I have no children of my own, I feel the terrible dread of losing a child. I try to shake it off but can't.

The physician's words bring me back. "How long has it been?" He checks the patient's pupils – fixed and dilated, a bad sign. The monitor has not changed.

We can't stop yet. He's too young. This is too senseless.

"Why don't we try temporary pacing? See if that works?" My suggestion is a desperate plea for more time.

The doctor looks at his watch. He knows it is futile, but shrugs. A nurse takes over bagging while I prepare the patient for an external, temporary pacemaker. I am hoping an electrical stimulus will fire up an impulse and then a heartbeat. It's a long shot, but I am at a loss. We have tried everything possible. I apply the pre-moistened gel pads, attach the wires, set the level of voltage and deliver the charge. We all wait for a response. Nothing. I raise the wattage. Still nothing.

"There's no use. It's been too long." The doctor runs his hand through his hair and leaves the room.

I glance over at the woman in the other room. Her eyes meet mine. *I am so sorry. If I could have willed his heart to start beating, if I could have laid my hands on him and healed him, I would have.* The woman closes her eyes, a single tear escaping.

Although we did all we could to save him, I am devastated. With a simple shift in consciousness, I experience this woman's feelings. I feel her pain and her helplessness. I feel her grief as if it were my own.

What do I do with emotions that aren't even mine to feel? I don't know how I am going to make it through my shift, to care for the patients I am assigned on the unit. Alone in the elevator, a sob escapes. I do my best to hold it all in, but tears stream down my cheeks. At my floor, I get off the elevator and slip into a utility room. I take big breaths of air and wipe my eyes.

Okay, suck it up. This is crazy. You have to keep going.

§§§

Trauma. A single defining incident that can change your life forever. It is experienced in the body as well as in the mind. In a flash the brain is rewired, thought circuitry disrupted, structures within the brain and the normal regulation of neurochemicals altered.

It is widely accepted that trauma can occur in victims of violent acts, rape, and life- threatening incidents. But it can also occur as a result of treating those victims and witnessing their suffering, regardless of whether that suffering is physical, emotional or relational in nature. Health care professionals are exposed to this almost daily. But since our focus is on treating the patient, little thought goes into how exposure to suffering may affect the caregiver. Common expectations such as "suck it up and carry on" or "this is what we signed up for" undermine the emotions experienced. We try not to think about it. We try and put it out of our minds. But in doing so, we don't process the thoughts and feelings as they should be processed. Traumas can be cumulative, with each additional incident affecting us more deeply until eventually the symptoms alter our lives significantly.

Largely subjective, what may traumatize one person may have little to no effect on another. Various factors such as previous exposures to traumatic events and how they were dealt with, individual coping responses as well as how resilient a person is will influence the degree to which someone is affected.

When I reflect back on this incident, I wonder what made it so different from the many other code blue situations I'd experienced. Normally the chaos of code blue consumed all my thoughts, yet in this instance I couldn't escape from a mother's distress. Were there other factors such as being overly tired, perhaps experiencing increased stress that made me more susceptible? These were questions that at the time I never knew to explore.

All I know is after this night, a change occurs in me. Instead of relishing the adrenalin rush of carrying the cardiac pager, I grow to dread it. The sound of a siren unnerves me. Death becomes my number one enemy. I am afraid of how I will react to another senseless death. My mind replays this incident over and over and over, and with it the intense feelings of grief. But I don't recognize the signs; I simply attribute it all to being part of the job.

Chapter 12

In the mid-1980s, cardiology was experiencing some groundbreaking advances in the treatment of myocardial infarctions, otherwise known as heart attacks. New drugs were being tested that dramatically affected patient outcomes. When I was working on the cardiology unit, antithrombolytics were the latest innovation. These drugs dissolve the clot that is causing the heart attack, and if administered within a certain time frame, can eliminate the damage done to the heart muscle. Our unit had completed the trials for one such drug called streptokinase, but a newer drug being trialled, TPA, was proving to be more effective and safer, with fewer possible complications like bleeding. Like many new drugs in research trial phase, TPA could only be used according to strict protocol. This regime included the presence of a research-approved physician, various scans and blood work and the administration of certain medications – all of which has to be completed within a very narrow time frame of the onset of symptoms.

One night shift, we admit a man in his mid-forties showing clear signs of a heart attack. Mr. Fortino is sweating profusely and is experiencing nausea and a crushing pain in his chest. His cardiogram shows ST elevation in the anterior leads, indicative of an anterior myocardial infarction, known as the "widow maker." Carefully, we transfer him from the stretcher to a bed, hook him up to the monitor and proceed to administer some morphine intravenously. I ask Mr. Fortino when his pain began. He explains that he called for the ambulance moments after it started. After going through a medical history, I know he meets all the criteria for TPA.

With wide eyes he grasps my hand tightly. "Please nurse, help me. I have two daughters your age. All I want is to see them get married. Please." He is frightened; he knows he could die.

I place my other hand over his and look him in the eye. "Mr. Fortino, we will do everything possible to make that happen."

Beneath my level of awareness, something inside has triggered. *I cannot let him die.* The monitor alarm goes off and I see a run of tachycardia, a sign that his heart muscle is becoming increasingly irritated with diminished blood and oxygen. After a few seconds, it returns to normal.

I leave him and approach the nurse in charge. "He's a prime candidate for TPA."

She nods and reaches for the TPA on-call schedule, determines which physician is on call tonight and dials the phone. I begin filling out some blood requisitions while I'm waiting. Flustered, she hangs up the receiver. "He said he is unavailable. We won't be able to do it."

"What? Did he say why? Can't he get a replacement?"

She shrugs her shoulders in defeat. I stand there blinking in shock. We have the tools to alter this man's outcome, but our hands are tied. *We can't lose him.*

"Let me call him back. This is ridiculous." How can we just stand by treating only the symptoms when there is a drug that will treat the cause?

I make the call and learn that after a gruelling day, the physician has just returned home. He isn't willing to come back in.

"Can we administer streptokinase if an emergency physician is available to stand by?" I am not even sure if streptokinase has been officially approved for use by the hospital administration. Every drug goes through various committees for approval, and last I heard it was still caught up in red tape. I wonder if what I am suggesting could jeopardize my licence to practice. I decide I don't care. There are a few moments of silence.

"Do I have the okay to administer streptokinase if I can get an emerg physician to be present?"

"Yes," he says finally, "as long as you don't need me to be there."

I hang up the phone. My blood is boiling. I go to write out the doctor's verbal order on the patient's chart and hesitate, knowing it would be inappropriate to record his words verbatim as I'm legally obligated to do. Hot anger rises within me. I am angry at having to give substandard care. I am angry at being put in this position. I pick up the pen and write, "May give streptokinase as long as you don't need me to be there." I sign the doctor's name and co-sign my own, then turn my attention to getting Mr. Fortino the help he needs.

I place a call to the nursing supervisor. As luck would have it, the one on duty is a former coronary care nurse. She gives full support to proceed. Racing against time and after a flurry of activity, we administer the drug.

Please, we can't lose him.

The beneficial effects are immediate and profound. Silently, I pray he has no untoward side effects, and fortunately he does not. By the end of my shift, Mr. Fortino is pain free and sitting up in bed, his cardiogram showing no signs of damage. *We beat Death.*

When I return to work after a few days off, I pass by Mr. Fortino's room. Sitting on the edge of the bed with his arm around one of his daughters, he smiles and gives me the thumbs up. I learn he underwent angioplasty as a precaution to ensure the patency of his arteries. He is expected to go home the next day. Relief swirls inside of me knowing how badly things could have gone.

On the unit, the director of patient care is waiting for me. Mr. Fortino's chart is open to the Doctor's Order page, to my entry made that night. I am reprimanded for my choice of words. I defend myself, stating that the words were verbatim. But this isn't good enough; I am expected to choose words that aren't so defamatory. There was no need to include "as long as I don't need to be there."

I know this to be true, but I am still angry about it all, how the patient could have died and how I was put in a precarious situation. I am encouraged to apologize. I leave the office certain that that will never happen and think if I had to do it all over again, I wouldn't change a thing.

When the anger subsides, all that is left is a sense of indifference. *What's the use?* I am tired of fighting the never-ending battle against death. I feel disillusioned, deflated. I carry on this way for a few months until I eventually decide a change of job is in order. During my twenty-two years as a nurse, I will change jobs eight times, unaware that I am searching for a job that isn't so emotionally volatile.

§§§

A common side effect of PTSD and STS is hypervigilance, an enhanced state of arousal that is often accompanied by an exaggerated intensity of behaviours. Hypervigilance may express itself in altruistic behaviour, as in my case. I had become a vigilante healer who would stop at nothing to achieve the means. It came with a cost: the possible loss of licence and the erosion of professional relationships.

A brain affected by trauma, primary or secondary, begins to see certain threats everywhere. My brain had sensed a threat. The posed threat wasn't just the possibility of losing a patient; it was having to face the family if we did. Everything changed for me with the mention of daughters. At that point, something shifted. I was going to do everything in my power to see that this man got the best care possible. I immediately assumed responsibility for his care. This is not how things are done. I had a full load of my own patients to care for and was merely helping out a co-worker when Mr. Fortino arrived on our unit. The nurse he was assigned to was more than capable of caring for him. But I just took over, even bypassing the nurse in charge. If my co-workers thought my behaviour "over the top," they never said. If the patient's outcome wasn't as positive as it turned out to be, maybe that would have changed things. For years, I believed my actions were right, never once recognizing what was really going on – that I was exhibiting a symptom of traumatic stress.

Hypervigilance is often accompanied by anger directed at those in authority. Even though I knew my actions were inappropriate, I recorded the doctor's order verbatim out of anger.

It would take years before I saw the situation with any degree of clarity and recognized another crucial lesson: as caregivers, we have to know and respect our limitations. For years I believed the doctor was wrong; that by agreeing to be a physician in investigative research, he had a responsibility to make himself available for his on-call shifts or find a replacement. But I think differently now. He simply understood his limitations and, by doing so, was able to have and full and rewarding career.

Chapter 13

I begin working for a community nursing agency. I plan my days according to the patients I need to see and the care they require. I drive around to patients' homes and welcome the freedom of no longer being confined to a building for twelve hours. The area I am assigned is a vast countryside that borders on cottage country. I start working there in the winter, and by spring I am surprised to see that the snow-covered fields, which I have driven by so often, are actually lakes. How great it is to stop for lunch at one of the many waterfront rest areas.

Many patients are regulars, like Mr. Murphy, the ninety-six-year-old potato farmer. He has lived his entire life on the family farm. When his brother and sister-in-law died, he sold it but retained the rights to remain in his small, wooden farmhouse located at the back of the acreage. The main house and its new family are within eyesight but far enough away for Mr. Murphy to maintain his own independence. The new owners take kindly to Mr. Murphy, driving him to his regular doctor's appointments and having him over every Sunday for dinner.

When I take over the care of Mr. Murphy, his regular nurse gives me an update on how he is doing. We are visiting weekly for a general health check and assistance with a bath.

"Don't let him talk you out of a bath! My bet is he'll do his damnedest at trying. It has been such a trial getting him to take a regular bath. And don't let him have the washcloth," she warned, "because he doesn't do a good enough job. You know, the first time I bathed him, I had to scrub his tub twice just to wash away the ring of dirt. It's a wonder he doesn't have lice!"

I take in all the nurse has to say. While the approach may have worked for her, I know myself well enough that I am not going to be able to pull off some militant air that will convince people to accept care. After all, it's not like hospital nursing, where patients are told what to do and when. No, this is different. I am a stranger in Mr. Murphy's home, and I feel that I need to respect that. He has every right to refuse treatment, even if it means jeopardizing his health. Somehow, I will have to find my own way of doing things.

As I knock on the wooden door of the old farmhouse, I wonder what homemaking horrors I will see. The door opens and a shy, elderly man stands waiting for me to explain the purpose of my visit.

"Mr. Murphy? I am the nurse scheduled to see you today."

"Oh," he mutters, and looks down at his feet. "I forgot you were coming."

Mr. Murphy does not appear ninety-six years old. He is slightly bent over but moves with good agility. His hair is white, and on his forehead is a distinct tan line where his hat likely sits. There is a smudge of dirt on his cheek, and the collar of his white t-shirt is lightly stained yellow. He brushes his hands on his twill pants, and I can see the dirt embedded in his fingernails.

We stand awkwardly at the doorway until he finally lets me in. The door opens into a room that serves as both a kitchen and a living room, the place where, when indoors, Mr. Murphy spends most of his time. An overstuffed sofa lines one wall, its floral fabric faded by sunlight. A small television stands on a table in the corner. A pine kitchen table sits in the middle of the room, with four mismatched chairs arranged around it. On the table is a plate, covered by another plate. I will eventually learn that after each meal, Mr Murphy simply scrapes any leftovers into the garbage pail, covers the plate with the other, and leaves it there ready to use for the next meal. As a bachelor, this is how Mr. Murphy handles clean up. For a moment I wonder if I should explain the assortment of ills one can get from improperly cleansed cooking utensils, but in the end I decide to postpone that conversation for another time and remind myself that Mr. Murphy hasn't lived to the ripe old age of ninety-six by sheer luck.

When I bring up the subject of a bath, Mr. Murphy apologetically declines and begins reciting a variety of reasons why it really isn't a good idea.

"I'm going out this afternoon and I don't want to get my hair wet. I'm not really sure there's enough hot water right now anyway. Besides, I gave myself a good sponge over last night."

I imagine what his previous nurse might say in response. *Oh come on now, Mr. Murphy, you know we need to get rid of all that dirt you have on you from digging up potatoes. Your skin is probably caked in perspiration. You know, don't you, that skin is the first line of defence to guard our bodies from infections of all sorts. It's so important to rid the body of dirt!*

Instead, I decide to take the time to get to know him a little better. I learn that Mr Murphy is a quiet man living a simple life. Most would think his life to be a sad and lonely existence, but he seems so content, so fulfilled. His days revolve around growing potatoes: hoeing, weeding, watering and eventually digging them up. Potatoes are the main staple of his diet as well as vegetables. I make a note to have his iron level checked.

As the weeks go by, on a few occasions there is no answer at the door, but I know enough to head around to the back of the house, where I find Mr. Murphy hunched over in the garden, tending his potato patch. Neat rows grow in uniformity, leaves lightly dusted to prevent his arch enemy, the potato bug, from getting to his crops.

The first time Mr. Murphy agrees to a bath, I turn the faucet on to fill the tub and add some liquid soap I keep in my bag. Soon the tub fills with bubbles. Then I leave the room, asking him to undress. After a few minutes, I knock and ask if he is ready. He mumbles and I enter the small cramped space. He stands naked holding his t-shirt strategically in front of himself, staring at the floor. I reach for a towel and wrap it around his waist, then assist him into the tub, removing the towel just before he becomes immersed in the shelter of soapy suds. He smiles as the warmth of the water surrounds him. Nicely concealed in bubbles, Mr. Murphy relaxes. Then I soap up a face cloth and give it to him.

"You go ahead and wash areas you'd rather do yourself, and I'll make sure your back gets a good wash."

He immediately starts to scrub down below.

After that first bath, Mr Murphy is much more at ease. Our relationship continues to grow over the weeks, and he even chuckles a few times.

One visit, after his bath, he asks if I know how to cut hair. I tell him frankly that I have never even trimmed my own hair let alone someone else's. But he persists, explaining that Sylvia, the woman who lives in the main farmhouse, is away and will not be able to take him to the barber until the following week. So I position him on a stool, close to the kitchen sink, where the lighting seems best.

"Are you sure you really want me to do this?"

"Yes, yes," he urges me on.

So with shears in hand, I slowly start snipping. Long pieces of hair fall to the floor as I trim his bangs, then around his ears, neck and back. Just when I think I am done, I stand back to look and see a small tuft of hair on the right side of his head, so I trim a little more. Then, of course, I need to even it up on the other side. Finally, I am done. I hand Mr. Murphy the mirror, rather pleased with myself. His eyes widen, and he throws his head back in surprise. After a few seconds, he smiles. "Well ... gosh ... sure is short! I guess I won't be needing another cut for a *very* long time."

Mr. Murphy never again asks me to cut his hair, but that is fine because he never again refuses a bath.

§§§

When I began working in the community, the level of acuity of patients at home did not compare to those I nursed in hospital. (The complexity of patients being nursed at home would grow exponentially in the years to follow.) Coming from a fast-paced, life or death job, I welcomed the change in environment. Community nursing gave me a much-needed breather of sorts. Although I was still exposed to death and dying, it was usually patients who were palliative and had chosen to go home to die, not those who had life abruptly stolen from them. Patients who know they have only a short time to live can prepare themselves and their loved ones, say what they need to say. For me, that type of exposure to death was easier to cope with.

Although a reduction in stress is beneficial for someone with STS, it is not a cure.

Chapter 14

A symphony of birds awakens me on Monday morning, and I look over at Bill and smile. On the weekend we got married. And since both of us have started new jobs, we decided it was best to postpone the honeymoon. There is too much going on. We bought a two-acre parcel of land outside the city that has fared well for both of us. We love it here. The sixty-foot trailer we call home is our temporary sanctuary as we build our house. Despite the cuts and bruises from framing, and scrapes on our knees from shingling, we are in heaven. But today is a regular workday and I must set aside my hardhat and tool belt and don my nursing cap, so to speak. Before we start our shifts as tradespeople, we have jobs to do.

I turn on the radio, and as I lay waiting to hear the forecast, I go over my list of patients. I'll start out with Mr. Casey; he needs his morning insulin. From there I'll head over to the Clarks'. Hopefully, with the change in meds, Mrs. Clark will be more comfortable. Of course, there's still the issue of her daughter. No pill can take away the pain of watching a loved one die. I'll have to make a point of pulling her aside to see how she's doing. With any luck, there will be enough time before lunch to do the initial assessment on the elderly couple who live on the outskirts of town.

"And so folks, don't forget your umbrella. With a sixty per cent chance of rain, my bet is you'll be needing it."

I shower, dress and grab some fruit for breakfast. Before I head out the door, I remember the weatherman's heed and ransack the closet for a large oversized umbrella.

A car pulls up beside me at a set of lights. Behind the wheel of a BMW sits a professionally dressed woman. We glance over at each other, and I can't help but wonder what it would be like to trade places with her for one day of corporate glamour. Nursing may be a lot of things, but glamour isn't one of them.

By 10:45 a.m., I am pleased with how smoothly my first three visits have gone. I pull over to the side of the road to review the referral sheet for my next appointment. *Eighty-four-year-old woman with Alzheimer's being cared for by her husband. Please assess level of coping.*

A few minutes later, I pull into the driveway of the small bungalow. Dandelion heads ready to disperse more seeds at the first hint of a breeze have taken over the front lawn. A tangle of branches from a large overgrown shrub spills onto the front walkway. I ring the doorbell and wait. A thin, scruffy tabby cat, eager for attention, rubs its neck on my pant leg. Finally, Mr. Knoff, appearing hurried, answers the door. I introduce myself as the community nurse who is scheduled to meet with him and his wife at eleven. He looks at his watch. He mumbles something about forgetting. An awkward moment passes, but when he realizes I am not offering to leave, he lets me in. I leave my umbrella by the door and he shuffles me down a dimly lit hallway and into the living room. Then he promptly asks if I would excuse him while he finishes assisting his wife.

I sit down on the couch and scan the room. The telltale clues of George and Sadie's existence emerge. A thick plastic sheet drapes the seat of an armchair. A cloudy glass of water with the settled remnants of a pill or two stands on the adjacent end table. Outdated newspapers are scattered across the coffee table, held in place by the crusted remains of a TV dinner.

I get up and approach the fireplace. A picture of a younger version of George and Sadie embracing graces an arrangement of family photos. Beside the photo of the couple stands an anniversary card. Yellow with age, it appears well worn, like a favourite novel that has been read over and over again. Memories of better years.

"I'm so very sorry to have kept you waiting," George's voice can be heard coming down the hall. "We're running a bit late this morning, had a bad night. I must have slept in."

George comes round the corner, gingerly ushering his wife into the room. Thin and frail, bearing little resemblance to the woman in the photograph, she clings firmly to her husband's arm.

"Not to worry," I said, "you've left me in good company." I glance down at the cat, and my pant leg, and the abundance of fur it has accumulated. This probably doesn't happen to that woman in the BMW.

I turn to Sadie, extend my hand to her and introduce myself. Making no attempt to take my hand, she eyes me suspiciously.

"Are you going to put me away?" she asks with a hint of defiance.

Flushed in the face, George pats his wife's arm. "Now, now, Sadie, you worry too much. We don't need to worry about that, do we?" His voice falters slightly as he speaks.

"No, Mrs. Knoff, I haven't come to put you away. I came to see if we might be able to offer you and your husband some help here at home."

George leads Sadie to the plastic-coated chair by the window.

"That's good ... that's good. That's good, isn't it George?" I watch as George puts her mind at ease with a smile and a pat on the arm. He lays a colourful crocheted afghan over her lap.

Completing the history and physical examination proves challenging. Sadie's memory is obscure, and she often seems detached from the conversation. Eventually, she drifts off to sleep, but not before George tucks a pillow at the side of her head. I am grateful for the opportunity to speak to George alone.

"So ... tell me George, what's it like for you?"

He pauses a moment and then glances back at his wife before speaking. "Sadie means the world to me. I have to do this for her." He swallows hard. "You know, I spent forty-five years driving a bus, and when I dreamt of retiring, I never pictured anything like this."

George goes on to describe his life, how he lives in fear that she will leave the stove on or wander outside at night. He admits to knowing very little about his wife's disease. But what he does know is that her condition has deteriorated significantly over the last year. She now needs help with even the most basic tasks: bathing, dressing, eating and toileting.

"Do you have any family, or friends?"

"Our son lives out of town and can't afford to visit very often. As for friends, well, it's hard for them too. The visits get farther and farther apart, until they stop coming around at all. I used to love the company."

"When was the last time you were able to get out on your own?"

"On my own?" George rubs his forehead. "Not for at least six months. I used to be able to leave Sadie at home while I ran an errand or two, but not anymore."

I sit for a moment admiring the courage and strength of the man before me. I appreciate the weight of his responsibility. It is the same weight that leaves me feeling heavily laden on many days. The difference being that George can't lay his burden down at the end of a shift, because his shift never ends.

"George, what keeps you going?" I have to know.

He thinks for a moment and sighs softly. "Well, it's all in how you choose to see things. Like when the weatherman says it's gonna be cloudy with a chance of sunshine, you can either believe it's going to rain, or you can hope for a little sun. Every day that Sadie knows who I am is a day of sunshine."

I lean over my bag, pretending to rummage through it for something ... anything ... just to give myself a moment. One of the most difficult things in life is to be the primary caregiver for a sick family member. Without outside support, the role can be all consuming. Responsibilities get juggled around, personal interests are put aside. With each passing day your own identity seems to slip away as you struggle to meet the needs of your loved one. And here is George, on his own waging a heroic battle against a disease that shows no mercy. *Collect yourself.* After a few minutes I feel able to speak. We spend some time going over a list of services that are available and together come up with a plan of care that will give George some much-needed help and even the opportunity to get out now and then. As I stand to leave, George speaks up.

"Thank you. For everything. I had no idea there was this kind of help. Just being able to talk about it with someone ... it was nice."

I take his hand in mine.

"Well you know something George? I think we both gained something from our visit today." I wink at him. "I've learned that I won't be needing *this*!" I wave the umbrella in the air.

In the car I make a note to follow up on Mr. Knoff. I think back over his words, but instead of feeling uplifted, I feel a dull ache. There is a duality in my life: the joys and excitement of starting a new life with Bill and the sadness of witnessing others struggle to hold onto theirs. I must learn to compartmentalize work and home in two separate areas of my heart. But that is tougher than it seems.

§§§

Developing secondary traumatic stress is a gradual, cumulative process. Often, as a defence mechanism, we try to discount our feelings. Traumatologist Anna Baranowsky calls this a "silencing response," which "guides the caregiver to redirect, shut down, minimize or neglect the disturbing information brought by an individual to the caregiver."[8] Changing the topic of conversation to avoid painful material, minimizing others' distress, becoming easily frustrated with patients, or having a difficult time being present – these are all ways to shield ourselves from further injury. And, whether we are aware of what we are doing or not, these behaviours are red flags that our defence mechanisms have gone awry.

Although defence mechanisms are usually in place to protect us, in a profession where caring is a fundamental tenet, these reactions can add to feelings of incompetency, guilt and shame as we recognize that our care lacks compassion.

Chapter 15

By my dates, my baby is almost three weeks overdue. So when the fetal monitoring begins to show signs of distress and there are no signs of going into labour, my doctor arranges for a C-section. Our first son, Michael, is born in February 1991.

We finished the house the previous summer (do you ever actually finish a house?) and had plenty of time to decorate the nursery for our bundle of joy. Or should I say our bundle of ongoing concern? Michael is a gorgeous baby who unfortunately requires very little sleep. As a new and naïve mother, my days are filled with entertaining him. I cherish this time with him, and so when my maternity leave comes to an end, I decide to go back to the hospital setting. I can't bring myself to leave Mike at a sitter five days a week as I would have to do if I remained a community nurse. If I go back to the hospital, I can work weekends while Bill is home, and I can be with Mike during the week. It will mean moving to more affordable housing, but I believe it is worth it. I am hired at a rural hospital within twenty minutes of our home.

Working for a small community hospital proves to be vastly different from my experiences at large urban centres. City hospitals pride themselves on being up to date on the latest technological advances and treatments. Day or night, all members of the health care team can be accessed. Hundreds of people work in a variety of positions. Because you rotate through shifts, there are always staff who are new to you. Such is not the case in a small rural hospital.

Rural hospitals see a diverse group of patients. The less critically ill are either treated in the emergency department and sent home, or admitted for further treatment. When a critically ill patient comes in, life-saving medical treatment is initiated, attempts are made to stabilize the patient, and then the person is transferred to a primary care centre. I had been used to having a team of people present to assist in those life-threatening situations. Not anymore. On many night shifts, it is quiet. Sometimes all it takes is a little health teaching and some basic nursing care. Once the last patient in emergency is taken care of, the physician on call might go home to bed or catch a nap in the doctor's lounge. But when major trauma victims are brought in, we are thrown into the race against time to save a life.

Working on the medical unit is a little more laid back. It is located on the second floor of an old two-storey building that accommodates about forty patients. Despite the age of the building, it remains meticulously cared for. The thickly waxed floors are buffed to a gleaming shine. The hot water radiators hum and hiss on the coldest of nights, sending clinking sounds through the thick cement walls up to the ceiling. Most nights are quiet. After the evening care is done and the hallway lights dimmed, patients sleep surprisingly soundly.

On the nights that patients settle well, we gather together in the staff lounge where we can readily hear any requests for assistance. Some knit or embroider amid the quiet chatter of our voices as we share pieces of ourselves and our lives. We laugh, we cry, we comfort each other, providing the sustenance to carry on in a multitude of life circumstances.

By 2:00 a.m. every night, we are ravenous. Sometimes a slice or two of pizza does the trick, other times it's nachos and dip. We often come well equipped for the night shift with an impressive spread of food to feast upon. When things are busy we nibble in bits and spurts, but when it's quiet we linger over these culinary delights. Eating a meal at that hour helps to ward off the waves of nausea that are sure to come by 4:00 or 5:00 a.m. That is the evil hour, the time of your shift when all bodily perceptions – stinging eyes, heavy limbs, giddy sensations – have to be ignored.

Around six in the morning, the smell of toast wafts through the vents from the kitchen below. A cosy feeling accompanies the smell of toast. Soon the shift will be over, and I will at last crawl into my own bed and heed the call of sleep.

To this day, the smell of toast makes me want to lie down.

§§§

It has long been understood that having positive social support has many health benefits. People still experience stress, but they do so with less physiological strain, and they are generally happier. Being part of a community fosters a sense of belonging and increased self-worth. Without social support, the obstacles we face in life become more trying. Having family or friends who understand your trials can be a lifesaver.

It is often difficult to speak with family about work-related experiences. Unless they are in health care as well, they will likely not be able to understand what you are going through.

But friends and acquaintances from work can and often do make great sounding boards. Strong social support networks are crucial, especially during stressful periods of life.

Chapter 16

Bill and I know from the moment of conception; no bells, no whistles, just an inner knowing. We are thrilled, and Mike, who is nearly two, is captivated by the prospect of being a big brother. If we are out shopping and I buy him a small toy, he insists on getting one for the baby. Although we are still in the midst of renovating the small lakefront home we moved into not long after my decision to go part-time, we are happy. With a new birth pending, I find myself wondering about the cycle of life and death. A person dies, a baby is born and the cycle of life goes on.

*

Harold is not expected to make it through the night. But he does. For two weeks the doctors keep telling his wife, "Mrs. Jenkins, it could be any time now." For two weeks she sits vigil at his bedside, taking over the role of gently swabbing his mouth with glycerine and applying Vaseline to keep his lips from cracking. An intravenous line, inserted to prevent the discomfort of dehydration, is all that sustains him. At times he awakens briefly from his morphine-induced sleep. She sees his eyelids flutter and is at his side in an instant with soft, soothing words telling him how much she loves him. Occasionally, he'll murmur in response, but most times he just squeezes her hand with what little strength he has left to muster.

Visitors come and go, not expecting to return. But they do, and the awkwardness of having to say goodbye again makes it all feel so painfully slow. It is taking a toll on Mrs. Jenkins. Dark circles hang under her eyes. Her clothes are wrinkled from having slept in the reclining armchair in his room. In situations like this, you don't just care for the patient. We begin taking note of Mrs. Jenkins's basic needs: is she eating, is she getting enough rest, is she coping?

And then Harold's breathing pattern changes, alternating from rapid and laboured breaths to intervals of nothing. The medical term is Cheyne Stoke respirations, also known as the "death rattle." "It won't be long now," the doctor says. But still he lingers on.

Two days later, after turning Harold over onto his side, I routinely check his skin for any evidence of pressure sores. To prevent skin breakdown, we would need to turn him every two hours, which would cause more pain. Since our biggest priority is comfort, we opt to turn him less often, running the risk of developing some pressure areas. Instead we place sheepskin covers under all the bony prominences of his gaunt, skeletal frame.

I go back to the nursing station with Helen, the nurse who has helped me with Harold's care.

"You know Helen, I'm not so sure that anyone can ever really predict when someone is going to die."

"Yeah, I know what you mean. Remember the woman in Room 211? She hung on for weeks and then died the day after her wedding anniversary, like she was willing herself to live until that day."

"Or patients who seem to hang on until their long lost son from out of town arrives," I add.

No, there has to be more to guestimating the imminence of death than judging by physical symptoms alone. How much influence does the human spirit have on its own release from life? Can people somehow decide how long to hang on or when to let go?

Mrs. Jenkins approaches the desk, relieving me of thoughts that I know can't be answered in this lifetime.

"A friend of mine came in to visit me, and since Harold looks so comfortable right now, I thought maybe we'd slip out to get a sandwich."

I look at her tired, pale face. How much longer can she endure this?

I nod at her and return to the notes I am making in Harold's chart. Once again, I begin thinking. What if it is actually possible to will yourself to "hang on" for a certain time? Then wouldn't it also be possible to "let go" at a certain time? A sinking feeling grows in the pit of my stomach. I hurry down the hall to Harold's room, passing Helen.

"What's up?" she asks, puzzled by my alarmed expression.

I don't stop to answer. I open the door and am relieved to hear the gurgle of a breath. I walk over to the bedside, waiting. One more breath, come on, she'll be back soon. But there is nothing. I clasp my hands around his and wait. Still nothing.

Helen approaches the bed. "Is he gone?" She takes the stethoscope from around her neck and places it over his heart, listens for a few minutes, then turns the intravenous off.

Just then his wife returns and reads the expression on our faces.

"No, *no!*" she screams. "I was just gone for a few minutes!" In desperation, she turns to me. "How could you let me go when you knew he would die? How could you?"

Her words cut like a knife through me. She breaks down in sobs. I reach over to comfort her.

"Please know, if I knew, if anyone of us knew, we wouldn't have let you go." But my words do little to comfort her.

After Mrs. Jenkins leaves the ward, the physician, who specializes in palliative care, comes in to pronounce Harold. Dr. Barter is well respected and known for his compassionate, caring ways. He is a natural in dealing with patients and their families. I know I can talk to him.

I sit down beside him. He looks up from the note he is writing.

"I feel awful. Harold's wife told me she was leaving, and while she was gone, he took his final breath. She was so upset with me for allowing her to leave."

Dr Barter puts down his pen. He looks at me, and I know he understands what I am feeling.

"I wouldn't have let her leave if I believed he was going to die while she was gone."

He nods. "I always tell my patients' families that death is a process. It is not as important to be there for the final intake of breath as it is to be there for the process. And she was there for the process."

I wish I had had those words when I was trying to comfort her. But I didn't. I wonder about sending her a note. I wonder about a woman who might go through the rest of her life believing she wasn't there for her husband, when she really was.

Something still plagues me. What are the chances that a woman who is vigilant about being at her dying husband's bedside misses the opportunity of being there for his final moments? In the last two weeks, she left the room only a handful of times. How could the moment of his passing happen just after she leaves?

"Do you think there is any chance that Harold could have been waiting for his wife to leave the room?"

Dr. Barter thinks for a moment, taking in a deep breath. "I think so. I really do. Sometimes patients want their family present. And others want them spared."

I shake my head. Hunches, really, is all we can go by. Relying on the physical state of the body doesn't guarantee accuracy in predicting the imminence of death. There is so much more to it, like the will to live, or not.

Too many unknowns, too many things about death that cannot be answered in this lifetime. For now, I will need to switch gears and concentrate on life.

§§§

By the very nature of our jobs, health care professionals often see patients and their families at their worst. It is not uncommon to end up the target of their frustration and anger. Mrs Jenkins lashed out in her grief. Likely she didn't mean her words to be hurtful, and yet they were. It is always helpful to question whether the accusations or complaints of family members are valid. Maybe there is something we need to learn. But if the reaction stems from their own frustration and grief, as in Mrs. Jenkins case, then learning not take everything personally is important.

A healthy self-esteem will minimize feelings of resentment when patients or family members react negatively and point blame where it isn't deserved, often because they are experiencing tremendous hurt themselves. It will also help in recognizing when a job is done to the best of your ability, regardless of what someone with less knowledge of the situation may think.

I am not speaking of verbal abuse or aggressive tendencies in patients, as those require action. Violence in the workplace is a reality in health care. Health care professionals are at the highest risk for being attacked at work, even when compared to prison guards, police officers, bank personnel or transport workers.[9] Many hospitals and organizations have instituted "zero tolerance" for any act of violence, whether it is physical, verbal, emotional or sexual harassment, and have dedicated resources to prevent and deal with violent situations.

Chapter 17

While Matt is napping, I engage Michael in the hunt for a lost item in the basement. I haven't seen my crepe pan since we moved. Since the kitchen is tiny, many of my small appliances remain in boxes. We have started renovations, but since Bill is doing most of the work himself, I suspect these items will be in storage for a while yet. We start opening boxes.

"Here it is!" It's become a game to Mike, and he wants to be the one to find it. Beaming, he holds up a coffee grinder.

"Hey, I was wondering what happened to that. Good work doll! But it's not a crepe pan." Mike looks pleased with himself anyway.

I open a box and find a cookie tin. It says *Butter Cookies* and has a picture of a chateau in the mountains on the top.

Mike sees it, his eyes widen, "Is that a castle?"

I remove the lid and hand it to him, my gaze falling on the contents of the biscuit tin. From early on in my career, I have collected items I consider *accolades*. In this box are thank you notes from patients or relatives, a letter written to administration by a doctor who took the time to commend my services, and newspaper clippings of public acknowledgements in obituaries. It serves as my little box of "feel good" reminders, a place to go whenever I doubt the impact of my actions. There aren't a lot of items, but many of my accolades don't have anything tangible that can be stored in a box. Instead they are stored in my memory.

*

The emergency department is busy. Since the med-surgical floor is quiet, I am asked to help out in the holding room, an area where patients stay while waiting for admission to the ward.

There are six stretchers filled with patients with a variety of ailments. At the far end of the room is Hilda, well known by staff because of frequent visits due to overexposure. Hilda is a bag lady. The smell of cheap wine filters the strong stench of bodily odour, prompting the patient beside her to ask if the curtain could be drawn more tightly.

"Hilda, how are you? It's been awhile since I've seen you."

Hilda glances up at me, tilting her head back to focus. There is little chance she remembers me.

"Did anyone get you something to eat yet?"

"Oh, a hot bowl of soup would go mighty fine right about now." Hilda brushes a long strand of greasy hair from her eyes. This action startles a few lice into jumping across the part in her hair. I take a step back.

"And after your soup, how about we get you into the tub?"

I walk away grateful for the warning, not like the time when I was a student and had the misfortune of unknowingly caring for a patient who had scabies – not an experience I am willing to repeat. Just the thought of it makes me itchy.

After Hilda voraciously consumes her soup and a sandwich, I don a hair net, an isolation gown that leaves me covered from my neck to my feet, and of course gloves. I help Hilda onto a commode chair and wheel her into the tub room that I have prepared for her.

Hilda is capable of washing herself so I sit on a chair by the tub waiting to help shampoo her hair.

"You know Hilda, it doesn't have to be this way for you." I thought I'd make another attempt at convincing her to accept some help. "We could arrange to find a place for you, you know."

"Oh no, nurse. You know me, there ain't no way anyone is gonna get me to go to one of those homes. I like my freedom. Ain't no freedom in those kinda places."

I go over to help her shampoo. With arms outstretched, I hold her head as she immerses herself in the warm soapy water. Lathering up with the medicated shampoo, I apply it to her hair as she hums a tune that sounds vaguely familiar. But I can't remember where I've heard it. As I massage the shampoo into her scalp, I can feel the small bumps from lice bites. When we are done, I help Hilda into a hospital gown and housecoat. Then I begin to comb through Hilda's hair with a fine-toothed comb. Carefully examining her scalp, I feel satisfied that the critters are gone. If we can convince Hilda to stay long enough, this treatment should be repeated in a few days. When we return to the holding room, I quickly strip her bed of all previous linen and place it in a doubled plastic bag, specially marked to warn the laundry staff. The many layers of clothing Hilda has been wearing go into another specially marked bag.

After I settle Hilda back onto the stretcher, I place a flannel sheet from the warming cupboard over top of her. She sighs heavily and glances up at me with a smile.

"Can I give you a hug?" she says, unsure of herself.

"Sure." I laugh and place my arms around her, grateful she asked now and not before her bath.

After a moment, I pull away. I look at her, pleased with how clean and comfortable she appears. She begins humming again, and now the tune comes to me. It is a hymn I learned as a child based on Matthew 25:40: *Whatsoever you do to the least of my brothers, so you do unto me.* Suddenly her image changes. I no longer see a pale, elderly woman with dark circles beneath her eyes, I see the face of a man, the face of Christ. I blink my eyes and the image is gone.

§§§

In the years to follow, whenever my job weighed heavily on me, I would sit down with the Saturday edition of the classifieds, bulging with opportunities for career changes. But my hopes would dwindle when very few of them could match the decent income I was making as a nurse, an income we relied heavily upon. During those times I would inevitably think back on this incident and wonder if maybe being a nurse was what I was meant to do. Maybe it was my purpose in life – a "calling" – something that I needed to accept.

For many people, spirituality is a wellspring of support in the face of difficulty. Prayer has always been a big part of my life, and although there were many occasions I gained a sense of solace through prayer, I have to wonder if religious beliefs can impose additional stressors – self-imposed expectations to carry on or to accept suffering as God's will. Witnessing the suffering of others and developing STS can inflict a spiritual crisis, a dark night of the soul. Speaking to a priest, pastor or minister might have been helpful, but without knowing what I was experiencing, and without the words to express what I was feeling, I was at a loss.

Chapter 18

When you live in a small town, everyone knows your business. The same holds true for working in a small community hospital. It's not that people are nosy; you just work so closely together that it becomes natural to share things about your personal life. Unless you're like Lynn, a nurse on our unit who worked diligently at keeping her private life off bounds.

When I think of Lynn, a tall imposing fortress comes to mind. One with large metal gates that slam shut with a loud clang and the clicking of padlocks. Lynn shares very little about her life and always remains on the fringe of our conversations. We make every effort to draw her in, but only on rare occasions do we get a glimpse of her real life. It takes months for Lynn to share with us that her mother-in-law, who has advanced Alzheimer's, has moved in with them. Lynn's personal life is a deep, dark secret, and we respect her right to privacy.

She doesn't need to reveal anything about herself for us to know she is a good nurse. Lynn is competent, caring and well liked. I watch her deal with a family who is being difficult, taking issue with the lack of their mother's progress, blaming anything from the medications to the prescribed treatment protocol.

Calmly, and with great respect, Lynn takes the family aside. Although I do not know what she says to them, I do know that when their meeting is over each of them embraces her, thanking her for all that is being done for their mother. Lynn soothes ruffled feathers with soft-spoken words. People know that she is listening. Lynn exudes compassion.

One afternoon, shortly after one of Lynn's terminally ill patients dies, she leaves the unit for a break, returning with reddened puffy eyes. I want to comfort her, let her know I know how she feels. But I don't. Because when I approach her the metal gates of Lynn's fortress slam shut and I don't feel it is my place to knock and be asked in. I am sorry that I didn't.

Not long afterwards, we begin to notice changes in Lynn. Occasionally she seems less inhibited, sharing snippets of information about caring for her mother-in-law. Other times she is quiet and reserved at the beginning of her shift only to seem giddy by the end of it. We all notice her mood swings, but when she starts to become distracted, our concerns for her increase.

It is around this time that we start to notice that narcotic counts are occasionally incorrect. It is standard policy that a nurse from the oncoming shift counts narcotics with a nurse that is finishing her shift. The narcotics are kept under lock and key, and any discrepancy warrants investigation.

At first, it is a single Dilaudid tablet that can't be accounted for. Then a couple of Tylenol #3 go missing. Then another nurse reports that the remainder of the contents of the morphine vial she had stored in the narcotic cupboard is missing. Little did any of us know, a full investigation was already underway with suspicions that one of the nurses was stealing a variety of different narcotics. A few days later, Lynn is suspended.

We are all shocked. Substance abuse is often a desperate effort to mask some kind of pain – physical or emotional. Was the wear and tear of caring for her mother-in-law on top of a career as a nurse too much for Lynn? None of us knew her well enough to know.

A few weeks later we are told Lynn is in rehab. A few people leave messages for her or send cards, but none are answered. We never see Lynn again.

*

It is late, close to midnight. I am tired but long for a few minutes alone. I have grown accustomed to this special time late in the evening, when the day's events replay freely like an echo in my mind. I tiptoe into both boys' rooms, relieved that sleep has lured them into a peaceful oblivion, and then to my room to find my husband deep in sleep, too. At last, the day is my own.

I reach for my cardigan and pull it tightly around me. I check its pocket satisfied that my *stash* is there, a crinkled pack of cigarettes. Passing through the kitchen, I pour myself a glass of wine – just what I need to take the edge off the day.

I open the back door carefully, hoping it will not creak, and step out into the chill of the late night air. It is early spring, and the crickets are in full symphony. I settle myself in a patio chair, carefully placing my wineglass on the table. I pull out the pack of smokes and light a cigarette, inhaling deeply. My head spins for a minute, but as I exhale I feel the tension give way. Muscles begin to unwind, a sense of calm comes over me and I close my eyes in relief. When I open them again I am aware of the stars. Tiny shimmering lights scattered across the pages of my life. I take a sip of wine.

An addiction has a way of fooling you into believing it can soothe some of life's greatest hurts. It does for me every evening. And for this reason, I dare not judge anyone like Lynn. Sometimes I find myself fooled into relief that it's not substances like narcotics or booze that have caught me in their snare. But then I come to my senses knowing that I am no less an addict, chained to a substance that I believe keeps me going.

Alone on the deck, I am free of my shame. It is just me and the stars that know my secret. No one here to look at me accusingly like I should know better because I am a nurse ... because I am a mother ... because. I know all of that. A wounded soul will seek solace in the strangest places and I seem to cling to the security of a crumpled pack of smokes.

Was it like that for Lynn? What reality was she trying to escape? Was the burden of caring for her mother-in-law, compounded by the stresses of her job as a nurse, too much? Addictions are often one of the maladaptive ways people choose in coping with their stress, their pain, their grief. Unfortunately, it is not uncommon for health care professionals to be caught in the same snare. A physician comes in, his words slurring. An obese social worker reaches for food every time the job becomes too taxing. A nurse goes outside for a smoke.

I inhale. I love this time, when thoughts are allowed to wander uninterrupted and insights settle over me like a mist blanketing the grass. I hear an owl hoot in the distance. This is my time. I have my little ritual to thank. Otherwise, there is no way I would make time for myself. How can something so soothing be so bad for you? How can something that is keeping me going be killing me? In the distance I hear a sound and strain to hear.

It's a bird's trill that sounds more like *Really?*

Simply knowing better is often not enough.

§§§

It is estimated that twenty per cent of practising nurses have issues with substance abuse and addictions.[10] Although the numbers are similar for the general population, risk factors for abuse increase in health care professionals as they frequently have easier access to controlled substances. Some hospitals have started random drug testing.

Addictions cause tremendous guilt and shame, probably more so for health care professionals. Having an addiction can be a breach of professional ethics and can put patients at risk. Developing healthier, safer ways of coping takes a lot of difficult internal work and time. The tendency towards addictive behaviours can increase when a person is experiencing STS.

Chapter 19

I stand at the end of our dock overlooking the lake. Homes dot the shoreline as far as the eye can see. A pontoon playing loud music heads toward town. The wind picks up forming ripples, then small waves. It feels like a change is in the air. I look back at our home. The 600-square-foot cottage we bought a few years ago has been transformed, thanks to Bill's hard work, into a 1,800-square-foot home. The last few years have been so busy with renovations, two small children, and the completion of my post-diploma nursing degree. We are happy, but something inside tells me we won't be here much longer. A few weeks later, Bill receives a job offer that is too good to pass up. It means relocating to a town more than two hours away. Since Mike is just finishing kindergarten, it seems like an optimal time to move. Bill's career as an engineer is beginning to take off and his opportunities for advancement are far greater than mine, even with my degree. It is an exciting time: an opportunity to improve our financial status, buy a larger home and even save for a cottage as we always dreamed of doing.

It is summer when we move, and I spend the next six months getting our family settled into our new lives. Even though the kids are young, the move proves to be a major adjustment for them. I spend most of my time trying to help them make new friends and volunteering in their classrooms. My presence is enough to give them the confidence to be themselves, and from there, making friends comes naturally. When I am comfortable that things at home are stable, I start looking for employment, eager to put my newly-acquired degree into use.

During the last phase of my program, I did a clinical placement at a home care agency and enjoyed the role of case manager. It was nine to five, weekends off, in a comfortable office setting. The job involved assessing, setting up and coordinating a variety of services for patients in their homes. Their needs ranged greatly from straightforward assistance with personal care to the treatment of complex medical disorders by specially trained health care providers who used highly technical equipment. Home care agencies employ a wide range of professionals as case managers – occupational therapists, physiotherapists, social workers as well as nurses – to pool the level of expertise and share each discipline's knowledge.

I enjoy working within a multidisciplinary team, and so I head off to the local home care agency. Within a few weeks I am called in for an interview. I am hired as a hospital-based case manager and begin work the following week. By all accounts, this seems like my dream job: one step removed from the frontlines, no more shifts, a clean office job. But if I thought it was going to be easier emotionally, I was wrong.

*

Three North is a medical unit bulging at the seams with elderly patients awaiting transfers to nursing homes, rehab units or home. Length of hospital stays are always under scrutiny, and physicians meet with stern warnings when patients exceed the average stay. Statistically, length of stay data reflect on a hospital's reputation and may impact funding. Added to that is the more pressing issue of patients in the emergency department waiting for a bed.

The urgency to get patients out filters down the line. So when I am assigned to Three North for the day, I know it will be hopping busy.

The day begins with a conference where we discuss every patient in the unit, focusing on who is ready for discharge. When we get to Edna Millie, the social worker explains that she is refusing to sign nursing home papers, stating that she wants to give "going home" another try. Weeks have gone by since Edna was admitted, and she has made little to no progress. Her lower extremities remain ballooned with fluid, increasing her difficulty in walking. She needs help with everything – transferring from her bed to a chair or a chair to the commode. She needs help with her meals and her personal care.

"Sounds like we need to precipitate an emergency," the doctor says, tapping his pen on his notepad.

"Excuse me?" I have no idea what he means.

"I said we need to precipitate an emergency."

"Yes, I heard you, I just don't understand what you mean."

"Well, it's apparent that Edna does not yet fully believe she needs the level of help that we all know she needs. Maybe a trial at home will convince her."

"You're kidding, right? The woman lives alone. Her family is out of town. She can't even walk." I look around the room. The other nurses, the social worker, the physiotherapist and occupational therapist are all staring down at their papers, unwilling to enter the conversation. I feel an annoyance growing at the ludicrous suggestion.

"Right then, let's set the discharge date for tomorrow." Then turning to me, he says, "You can get the services in place in time?"

I feel a wave a panic spread over me. "Services? I can't provide near the amount of services she needs, and you know that." My voice is defiant.

"Yes, I know, but that is what she needs to understand." He closes his notepad and prepares to leave.

I sit stunned. Edna is not ready to go home. I envision the ambulance attendants bringing her home, placing her in the recliner of her living room. The wheelchair I will have delivered will be out of reach, useless to her without the help of someone else, as will be the commode. I wonder if she will attempt to get up on her own, which would be dangerous. I decide that she won't, she can't, she still doesn't have the strength or muscle tone to lift those distended, swollen legs. She will sit and wait until morning when help will arrive. No doubt she will be sitting in a puddle of urine or feces.

I go straight to the phone to restart her home care services. Fortunately, they can send someone to be there shortly after she arrives.

"Make sure they leave her a sandwich or a snack of some kind within reach. And water," I add.

I place a call for our equipment provider, who assures me they can have the wheelchair and commode out by tomorrow afternoon.

I call Eileen, her community case manager.

"Eileen, you are not going to believe this. They are sending Edna Millie home tomorrow." My news is met with silence.

"I thought she wasn't getting any better."

"She's not any better, and apparently refusing to sign papers for a nursing home. So the powers that be feels she needs a wake-up call. I can't believe it."

Eileen and I started working for the community home care agency at the same time, and neither of us have ever heard of "precipitating emergencies." I tell Eileen I have timed a home-making visit for when she arrives home so they can set her up for the night, and then again in the morning. Edna does not qualify for the twenty-four hour care she requires because she is not terminally ill.

"Can you get out to see her tomorrow morning? And if you find her in quite the state, send her right back in?"

"You mean *when*, not *if*, I find her in quite a state."

"Yeah." I hang up and take a deep breath. I make it through the rest of the morning, but by the end of the day I am irritable, frustrated and just plain worried.

The next day, I go in to see Edna before she goes home. Cognitively, she's all there and for that reason she cannot be forced into a nursing home. She understands that to go home, she is placing herself at risk, but tells me that she still wants to give it another try. I go over the services she qualifies for, trying not to sound apologetic for not being able to give her what she needs. I am restricted by policies and criteria. Before I go, I ask if her phone is within reach of her chair. She assures me it is, and thanks me. I leave, feeling a great unease about this whole predicament.

That night, I awaken at 2:30 a.m. thinking of Edna. Is she hungry? Thirsty? Thoughts of her rob me of any possibility of sleep, so I get up and make myself a cup of tea. She has probably been incontinent by now, forced to relieve her bladder in the very chair she is sitting in. Even worse, maybe she has fallen. Maybe she is lying injured on the floor.

Should I go to her?

I know that if I do, I will feel relieved. I could help her onto the commode, help her out of her urine-stained clothing, place a pad down to protect her from the moisture. I could make sure she's okay. Refill her water jug.

But if I go, I will be sending her the message that help will be available. She will never get a visit in the night unless she hires help privately, and financially that isn't a possibility. No, my help will only confuse her and delay the obvious decision that needs to be made. A decision that only she can make.

I go back to bed and spend a fitful night tossing and turning.

At 9 a.m. my pager goes off. It is Eileen. She has called an ambulance to have Edna brought back in.

"How is she?"

"Exactly where the ambulance drivers left her. Honestly, she's not any worse for wear, except for a really strong stench of urine. But she does seem a little defeated. And she's ready to sign those papers."

§§§

Health care providers face ethical and moral dilemmas like this one every day. Sometimes the issue is the unnecessary prolonging of life, other times we feel that not enough is being done.

For the longest time I felt frustrated, angry and ashamed whenever I thought of the incident with Edna. I didn't want to play any role in it. And what about the oath I took to do no harm?

These situations can eat away at you, or you can choose to see things differently. The doctor who spearheaded Edna's "medical emergency" understood something very important: compassion may necessitate an unconventional approach. Something akin to tough love. He could have taken away Edna's right to make the decision to go home, forcing her into a nursing home where she would likely have spent the rest of her days feeling embittered and frustrated, like a victim who has lost all control. But he didn't. He allowed her to come to the decision on her own, thereby maintaining her dignity.

But I remained at odds with this situation, like my brain and heart were unable to resolve their opposing opinions. The distress of situations like this intensifies the symptoms of STS. The whole scenario plays over and over again in your mind, and each time the body responds with its flood of cortisol and its redirection of blood flow to essential organs. Tolerance diminishes and coping becomes more difficult.

Chapter 20

During the summer, the boys like to plan my days off. A long bike ride is often first on their list, so when I suggest we pack a picnic lunch, the boys cheer at the prospect of making a day of it. There are an abundance of parks in the area, but we decide to hitch up the bike rack and drive the short distance to Niagara-on-the-Lake to take advantage of the long meandering bike path that leads to Niagara Falls. I'm guessing that would be around twenty kilometres, round trip – too far for a six- and eight-year-old, too far for me. But how far we get is not the point. What's important is the adventure and the time we spend together. It's about making memories.

We park at Fort George National Park and unleash the bikes from their restraints. The boys are bubbling over with excitement. With backpacks strapped in place we head along the paved path, leaving the quaint town behind. Soon the path winds its way beside the well-manicured lawns of upscale homes backing onto the river. The boys ride in front as I go at a slower pace, taking in the sights. Before long, the residential area gives way to vast stretches of greenbelt. It feels as if we are in the countryside. We ride like this for ages, sometimes in single file, sometimes chatting side by side. I am loving this moment – the broad grins, the sun-kissed cheeks and the laughter.

After some time, I glance at my watch and realize that a few hours have gone by and it's time to refuel our bodies. We come upon a roadside fruit stand with plump red cherries for sale. I buy a quart, perfect for dessert. We find a great spot to sit and have lunch, a shaded grassy area next to the woods lining the bank of the river. We can hear the water from where we are sitting. Although it is warm out, there is a pleasant breeze keeping us perpetually fanned. I check the boys for signs of wear and tear: nothing, not surprising. We devour the sandwiches, surprised at how hungry we are. I am relishing the break from pedalling, and to prolong our rest period I get the boys involved in a cherry pit-spitting contest. First we plunk the ripe cherries in our mouths, the juices squirting with the first bite. Then we carefully eat the pulp, position the pit between our lips and blow with a mighty force. We're aiming for deep within the wooded area. We are laughing about coming back to this very same spot in a few years only to discover a cherry tree orchard, all because of us.

Suddenly a wave of fear comes over me. That's what it feels like – fear. My body has grown tense, my stomach is knotted and my heart begins to race. At first I'm not sure why, but finally my senses catch up to my subconscious. I am reacting to the sound of a distant siren, the faint but unmistakeable sound of an ambulance. I look around, unable to determine its location. It isn't loud enough to be close.

I am in the emergency room of the small rural hospital where I used to work. It is late at night. Ambulance dispatch has called letting us know an ambulance is on its way. There has been a car accident out on County Road 6. We are told the age, gender and status of both victims. We are told brief but necessary details about the accident: head on, both belted. Details that foretell the type and severity of injuries we should expect. We phone the on-call physician who previously left because the night had been quiet. He will arrive in minutes. We are on high alert, adrenalin already pumping as we prepare the trauma room with equipment like IV bags and tubing, oxygen masks and endotracheal equipment.

"Mom?"

"Mom, you're not listening." Michael turns my face to his. *What had he been saying? What did I just miss?* I no longer hear the siren.

"Oh I'm sorry, hon. I was just thinking about something. What were you trying to tell me?"

Michael slumps down beside me, dejected. This is not the memory I had hoped to make. How often in their lifetime will my children try to get my attention only to discover that their mom is lost in thought?

I reach over and tickle him, coaxing him to tell me what he had wanted to say.

Eventually, between fits of laughter, he lets me know that one of his cherry pits flew so far that it landed by the bank of the river. Now that he has my attention, he is back to feeling proud. With only a few cherries left, Matt and I do our best to beat the new target, but the wind has picked up, preventing the pits from flying too far. When all the cherries are polished off, we crown Mike the king and Matt the prince of cherry pit spitters and head off for home.

§§§

Families and friends of people with Secondary Traumatic Stress often have to live with its side effects. Dealing with erratic mood swings, distancing or the distractions of loved ones suffering from STS can be difficult, and probably more so when the cause of those side effects isn't known. Issues of intimacy between spouses can develop. Longstanding friendships can become estranged.

A few years ago, I had a conversation with a young woman who was deciding what career path to follow. She explained that her mother was a social worker, and when I asked if she was considering a similar path, she was adamant she was not. "My mother didn't have a whole lot left to give us kids when she got home from work," was her response.

A vacant parent. An unresponsive partner. We owe it to our families to gain a better understanding of STS and how it affects not just our own lives, but the lives of those we love.

Chapter 21

Over the summer, the union is negotiating a new contract. Salary, seniority benefits and retirement plans are on the table. As the weeks pass, the rumblings of dissension grow. My co-workers complain about the "ill-treatment" they receive, the lack of respect and the "over the top" restrictions placed on them. I feel confused. In the short time I have worked at this home care agency, I have never been treated with anything but respect. As far as I know, the management team works diligently to address the concerns of staff members. But it seems to be a matter of interpretation. When all the office chairs are replaced with more ergonomically correct ones, I am grateful for managers' concern for our well-being. My co-workers, on the other hand, dismiss the initiative as having less to do with our well-being and more to do with minimizing absenteeism. By late summer, all negotiations have failed and talk of a strike looms. I speak up, questioning the timing of the union's demands; the provincial government is tightening purse strings. Did they believe they could get blood from a stone?

Until this point in my career, striking has never been a possibility. As an *essential service,* it was illegal for nurses to strike. Eventually, rotating strikes came into existence but never in an institution where I was employed. In the community, a strike was legal. It caused a great deal of upheaval within the health care system, with hospitals overburdened by additional admissions and management juggling caseloads of thousands. Patients would still get care, albeit haphazardly.

I brace myself for what I know will be difficult times. Since Bill is in management, I have an understanding of how ugly things can get. People behind the picket lines transform into people they normally aren't. Name calling and yelling obscenities aren't uncommon. Neither is aggressive behaviour toward anyone who wants to cross the picket line. A type of gang mentality ensues, and somehow society in general seems to accept that kind of conduct. What I find perplexing is that picketers believe their behaviour justified and expect that all will be forgotten when the strike is over. But I know from Bill that it is never forgotten.

A strike vote is called, and the results are nearly unanimous. Only a handful of us are against it, mainly those of us who have been recently hired. How can I take issue with a salary that, just six months prior, I agreed to? I did not opt into the retirement plan because I knew there was a good chance we would move again in another five years or so. The benefits that seniority provides are a non-issue for me as well.

In all my years as a nurse, I have always paid union dues. I appreciate the substantial impact unions have had on employee wages and benefits, and their pivotal role in issues of workplace safety and employee rights – and yet, timing is everything. With the newly-elected government significantly cutting budgets within the home care sector, I cannot see how the union's demands of a twenty per cent increase in wages, to reach parity with hospital salaries, could be successful.

When you belong to a union, and are in agreement with the mainstream of thinking, you appreciate the strength in numbers. But if you are in opposition, your voice is simply discounted. I feel as if I have no voice.

I am in a predicament. Should I rally behind my co-workers and head off to the picket line, even if it is against my convictions? If I don't, I will jeopardize the relationships I have made. Already, the concerns I have voiced against picketing have been met with cold stares of disapproval. Should I become a "scab," a traitor who crosses the picket line? In the end I choose the middle ground. I do not join the picket line, nor do I cross it. While my co-workers head off to picket, I remain at home searching the want ads and surfing the net for new employment opportunities. There is nothing within reasonable driving distance. After a few weeks, I am notified of a union meeting.

I enter the hall and immediately become aware of the chilly sideways glances and stares. When I approach a chair, one of the case managers quickly puts her purse on it. "You can't sit there." She rolls her eyes at the few others sitting at the table. A few people approach me and ask outright, "Why haven't we seen you on the picket line?" Their tone is harsh and condescending. During the meeting one person stands up and asks to address the issue of the *scum* who are choosing not to support the picketers. As she says this, she turns and glares at me. I sit there feeling the blood rise in my cheeks. When the general meeting concludes, I speak to some of the other newer employees who have been against the strike. I can see they are shaken up as well, and it looks as if their convictions are about to cave.

The next day, the unpredictable temperatures of November drop. I lay in bed knowing that in a few hours my co-workers will be heading off to the picket lines to endure the blustery winds and frigid cold. I cannot get their disapproving faces out of my mind. I pull the covers over my head. I feel that every ounce of courage has left me. Is it the courage to join the picketers that I need, or the courage to stay away?

Tidbits of information filter down to me regarding the incidents that occur on the picket line. A few people are trying to rally support for picketing the homes of any personnel choosing not to picket. One supervisor, who is deathly allergic to peanuts, is taunted by picketers waving a bag of nuts at her as she crosses the line each day. I become more convinced to stay away.

Days before Christmas, the strike ends. The small increase in salary pales in comparison to the loss of income after striking for twelve weeks.

I am unsuccessful at finding another job, and so I too return to work with the others. My presence is not well received. One co-worker pulls me aside and says, "What are you still doing here?" Another says to me, "Are you happy with the raise I got you?" A few others find small but irritating ways to make my job as difficult as possible. I no longer feel that I can tap into the resources of other health disciplines. When I enter a room, I am met with whispers and glares. In the cafeteria, I eat alone. I go in each day, do my job and then go home. For the first time in my life, I understand how it feels to be socially shunned.

§§§

In the 2005 National Survey of the Work and Health of Nurses, it is reported that forty-four per cent of nursing staff have been bullied at some point during their career.[11] The nursing profession has been accused of "eating their own." Bullying is a serious and growing problem that negatively affects the well-being of employees and the performance of organizations. Bullying behaviours can range from facial gestures to isolation techniques, to withholding information and refusing to work with or help a colleague.

The workplace culture needs to change. Organizations need to create policies to prevent workplace harassment and violence, and to educate their staff.

Those suffering from STS are particularly vulnerable to the pressures of bullying. If you are already having trouble coping, being bullied can make a difficult situation intolerable. The stress of being socially isolated, or worse, shunned by your co-workers intensifies feelings of insecurity and helplessness. Self-esteem diminishes as support systems that are fundamental to coping erode. Inevitably, a feeling of humiliation ensues.

Chapter 22

I open the employee directory and discreetly jot the number for the Employee Assistance Program on a pad of paper. After I leave the office, I place the call. A friendly voice answers. I freeze for a moment, not sure what to ask for, but eventually I manage to spit out that I would like to see someone. The friendly voice must be used to awkward calls like mine. She knows enough not to ask too many questions or she'll lose me. The questions she asks all pertain to things I'm willing to answer: name, address, place of employment. I hang up, grateful that she did not ask about the purpose of my visit. I don't know what I would have said.

On the day of my appointment, I park the car a block or two away from the address I've been given. I am early. As I approach the building, one of the supervisors from work is leaving. From the stories I heard, she endured a lot during the strike. We exchange embarrassed glances and pretend we did not see each other. I enter the building through a series of doors that are structured so that patients arriving will not see those leaving – a gesture toward confidentiality. A little too late for the supervisor and me.

In my haste to make the appointment, I realize I have no idea what qualifications the counsellors have. I end up concluding it doesn't matter; the counsellor will be from whatever agency the Employee Assistance Program contracts its services to.

I am ushered into a small office and the door closes behind me. The room is sparsely furnished – a desk and two chairs. There is no window. As I take a seat, a woman roughly my age knocks and enters the room. She wastes no time in asking why I am here. I tell her how awful my work environment is, and how since the strike I am disliked by most of my co-workers.

"I think they are out to get me – like they'd love to see me fail."

"Tell me more about why think they're out to get you," she says in a soothing, professional voice.

"Well, they're always whispering behind my back, and rolling their eyes when I walk past them, and giggling. I try to ignore it but I know it's directed at me. I don't feel that I can ask anyone for routine help. Like the time I received a referral from the intake department. I needed clarification on some of the information they put down, but when I went to them they laughed and said, "Do you really think I'm going to help you out?"

Just getting that off my chest makes me feel better, until the therapist's line of questioning goes in a direction I'm not comfortable with.

"So, you feel like everyone is laughing and talking behind your back?"

"Yes, I do," I answer.

"Hmm. Tell me, do you ever hear voices? Do you ever feel like you're being followed?"

Oh. My. Gosh. The woman thinks I'm paranoid, probably because I said "they're out to get me." I begin to see how that might sound, but I can't believe what is happening.

"Look, I know it seems a bit crazy. And it is, but not in the way that you may be thinking." I am defensive now. "I may be dealing with some stress issues, but I'm not paranoid."

She sees that her line of questioning has upset me. She changes the topic. We discuss ways to counteract stress – novel ideas like eating right, yoga, relaxation. At the end of our session, I thank her. She attempts to schedule another appointment, and I tell her I will have to call later as I don't have my date book. She seems satisfied with this and I leave, never to return again.

I go back to work. I drag myself in every day. As the months go by, new case managers are hired. Since they weren't around for the strike, I am able to make a few new friends. But by then I have made a point of distancing myself. It's my method of coping. It's called pretending. I pretend my co-workers reactions don't bother me, I pretend nothing bothers me. But every day that I go on with this facade, it's taking a toll on me.

Before long, physical symptoms of illness set in. I have a lump in my throat that won't go away. I am tired all the time. I am sleeping poorly at night.

At first I attribute my difficulty swallowing to my morning routine. To save time, I make toast and eat it while driving to work. Probably not a great idea because on the drive I battle a bundle of nerves. I try to remain calm and think positively, but inevitably I stew about it. The toast feels like sandpaper on my throat. I rinse it down with a gulp of coffee. When it reaches the point that I am constantly aware of this difficulty in swallowing, I arrange for a doctor's appointment.

After a slew of tests – x-rays, blood work and a barium swallow – the results come back inconclusive. I am referred to an ear, nose and throat specialist. He places a tube down my throat and sends me home with a clean bill of health. How could nothing be wrong when I feel like I've swallowed a golf ball and it has lodged in my throat? To top it off, after the barium swallow, I begin experiencing a burning sensation in my oesophagus. I am put on Nexium, a drug used to treat reflux and oesophageal ulcers. It has some effect on my throat but doesn't completely take away the discomfort.

The worse part of it all is knowing I am a sitting duck. I am under a great deal of stress. The source of my stress is my job. And I am trapped there until I find a new job or we move again. Already the head-hunters are calling Bill, whose expertise in manufacturing is well sought after. But it isn't happening fast enough for me.

So I start yoga classes, do breathing exercises and listen to a relaxation tape. I make sure to eat my quota of fruits and vegetables. I get away for a "girls' weekend" with nurses I used to work with, and laugh until my sides hurt.

I beg my body to hang on.

§§§

In his book *When the Body Says No*, Gabor Maté, MD, describes how stress transmutes into illness.

> Stress is a complicated cascade of physical and biochemical responses to powerful emotional stimuli. Physiologically, emotions are themselves electrical, chemical and hormonal discharges of the human nervous system. Emotions influence – and are influenced by – the functioning of our major organs, the integrity of our immune defences and the workings of the many circulating biological substances that

help govern the body's physical states. When emotions are repressed ... this inhibition disarms the body's defences against illness. Repression – dissociating emotions from awareness and relegating them to the unconscious realm – disorganizes and confuses our physiological defences so that in some people these defences go awry; becoming destroyers of health rather than its protectors.[12]

Somatization is the process in which emotional stress is translated into physical symptoms. The ailments are real, but their root cause is largely emotional and stress related. Stress-induced illnesses include migraines, backaches and gastrointestinal symptoms. Each individual's body system seems to have an area that becomes particularly vulnerable. Reflecting now on the difficulties I had with my throat, I can't help but wonder if it was associated with the loss of a voice, an inability to articulate what I was experiencing.

Chapter 23

I drop the boys off at the YMCA day care, kissing them goodbye in the car because they are too *old* to be seen kissing their mother in front of friends. I watch them head inside like troopers, knapsacks secured firmly on their backs. I think wistfully of the good ol' days when we would plan a day of leisure. But those days are gone, and I have a dreaded assessment to do. It's not just any assessment; it's an assessment to determine a patient's capacity to make a shelter decision. In plain English, I have to determine if my patient, Mrs. Topski, is *with it* enough to be able to decide to remain in her own home. If I deem her capable, she maintains the right to decide. If I determine that she is incapable, she can be forced against her will to go to a nursing home.

I pull onto the highway, going through my opening words over and over.

"Mrs. Topski, I am here to ask you a few questions. The questions will determine if you are capable of making a shelter decision. May I proceed?"

No, too formal and bureaucratic. The woman is in her eighties. I try again.

"Mrs. Topski, hello, how are you? How are things going for you here at home? I was hoping to ask you a few questions today, questions that will determine whether you understand the risks you face by living in your home alone. May I go on?"

Capacity assessments rank highest on my "hate to do" list, probably because I have no faith in my ability to do them properly. Not because I am incompetent, but because I believe that these assessments are beyond my skill set. In other parts of the country, this task falls into the hands of qualified professionals like psychiatrists or geriatricians, or a team of professionals that includes social workers, doctors, nurses and psychiatrists. Not just one solitary case manager.

I am told that this is the way it is. "You are merely doing a 'capacity to make a shelter decision'; it is not a competency assessment," as if I am making a mountain of a molehill. "Those are done by doctors." Those assessments include financial, medical and legal rights.

But to me, choosing one's home is still a fundamental human right, and one that I might be responsible for taking away. It's a big deal.

All the reading I have done on the topic does little to boost my confidence in my ability to proceed in a capable way. What nags at me the most is that often people will tell you what they think you want to hear, and downplay the risks they are actually facing. The whole process feels like a mind game with me trying to figure out if that's what they really believe or if they are just giving lip service.

The protocol I am to follow is explicitly clear. I must obtain permission before I begin asking the questions. Stories circulate through the office of case managers who were sued because they either failed to ask permission or proceeded with questions without explaining their purpose. It is a legality.

I arrive at the client's home by 9:00 a.m. I open her file and briefly read through it. I have not yet met Mrs. Topski because I took over a new caseload a few weeks ago. Her daughter greets me at the door. She has flown in from out of town in response to a call from her aunt. Family members believe it is time for Mrs. Topski to go into a nursing home. I spoke to the daughter a few days before, and was told that Mrs. Topski has been wandering the halls of her apartment building at night. The neighbours, all long-time residents, know her and take turns bringing her home. The stove was unplugged months ago as a precaution, and Mrs. Topski goes upstairs to her sister's for meals.

The daughter ushers me into the living room, where Mrs. Topski and her sister are sitting. I greet them, introducing myself.

"Mrs. Topski, I am here today to ask you a few questions." She stands up, points her finger at me and in a loud voice says, "I *know* why you're here. *You're here to put me away!*"

Mrs. Topski's sister, her daughter and I are all taken aback. I make an attempt to smooth things over.

"I would like to ask you a few questions to see if you are aware of the dangers or risks of living alone. Is that okay with you?"

"I want you to *get out!*" She moves across the room and sits at the dining room table.

I look at the daughter. There is nothing I can do. Her refusal leaves no doubt, nor does her comment about why I am visiting.

I explain to the daughter that I will not be able to proceed. She becomes angry. She has flown half way across the country for this meeting. How can I just leave?

I excuse myself to make a phone call to the office. I track down my supervisor, explain the situation, the client's resistance, the daughter's situation. I am told not to proceed. She has refused. That is all there is to it. We will have to find another way to deal with it.

By the time I get back to the office I have several messages from a nurse who works with the chief geriatrician at the hospital. I call her back. She already knows about the incident, the daughter has called her appealing for help.

"Oh, come on Dorothy. Clearly the lady is demented. Can't you see that?"

"Well actually, I don't know that. It was the first time I have met Mrs. Topski and in the short time I was there, she couldn't have been clearer."

That sets the nurse off. She goes over all the details the daughter has told me.

"I know all that, and I'm not saying she isn't demented, I'm just telling you that my hands are tied. She refused the assessment. I cannot proceed under those circumstances. And you know that, Ann, you were doing these assessments less than a year ago." Ann was a case manager who left during the strike to go work for the geriatrician.

I hang up. *You're here to put me away!"* replays in my mind like a broken record. It will continue to do so for days. What should I have done? Rephrase my question? I tried that. In the end, I don't know what I could have done differently.

By afternoon, I have several calls from various members of the health care team who know Mrs. Topski, wondering why I didn't proceed with the assessment. I try to explain the reason my hands were tied, why I was unable to proceed, but none understand the protocol involved in the assessment. To them, all I have to do is fill out a form.

The next day, I approach my supervisor. I feel terrible about the daughter's situation. "Any suggestions about what I should do about Mrs. Topski?" Even though the woman was very clear about knowing why I was visiting, the information I received from family does suggest there are issues. Would she benefit by going to a nursing home? Probably. Was she at risk? Probably, at least judging from family reports. I don't think she's in any imminent danger; she has strong support systems in place. Her sister and the neighbours have been caring for her in that way for months. Of course she could fall and break a hip, but she is no more likely to than anyone else.

"Okay, schedule an appointment for early next week."

I make an appointment with the daughter, the sister, Mrs. Topski, my supervisor and me for the following Tuesday. The date is September 11, 2001.

On Tuesday morning as I am preparing for the visit to Mrs. Topski's, a secretary comes by yelling that a plane has just crashed into one of the Twin Towers. We all gather around watching CNN Live reporting the tragic events going on in New York, and then Washington. I watch, horrified. This is the most tragic event I have ever witnessed. I want to leave work. I want to go pick up my children. I, like so many people in both the United States and Canada, feel the terrifying threat of a homeland invasion. Is this the start of World War III?

Shortly after the second plane tears into the second tower, my supervisor comes by ready to leave for our appointment. The horrifying images remain vivid as I drive. When we arrive at Mrs. Topski's home, she is glued to the television, watching the events unfold. My supervisor has no luck in obtaining permission either; Mrs. Topski shoos her away. "Can't you see how important this is?" she says. Another moment of clarity. My supervisor calls the client's doctor, who agrees to have her admitted to hospital where they can observe her and do an assessment from there.

I suspect that Mrs. Topski's admission won't go over well with hospital administration. It will be perceived as "passing the buck." Within a few days, the chief geriatrician arranges a meeting with all the case managers to discuss capacity assessments. I know it is no coincidence. It is my situation he wants to put on the chopping block.

I enter the meeting room feeling that I am entering a nest of vipers. The geriatrician begins by asking if anyone is having or has recently had any issues with doing capacity assessments. He poses the question in a cocky, taunting way.

I shift in my seat. *The bastard.* He knows darn well I have. He's putting out the bait in hopes I will take it. It's the last thing I want to do. I don't want to explain to a room full of unfriendly people what happened, to justify my position, to admit my self-doubts, my inadequacies. But I know if I don't, it will look worse. I stand up.

"Yes, I have, and I believe you are well aware of the situation."

He seems pleased. I have taken the bait. He looks at his nurse, the one I spoke with on the phone. They look as if they have caught the mouse in their trap. For the next hour, we discuss the issues of this case. I defend my actions, I argue against their suggestions. Eventually a few other case managers add their opinions, supporting mine. By the end of the hour I am exhausted. We don't come to any resolution. But the team from the hospital no longer appears cocky.

§§§

Stress and STS feed off each other. Stress is a contributing factor to the development of STS; STS reduces tolerance of stress. It becomes a vicious cycle. Soon, things that normally wouldn't cause tension become unbearable. Altered perception caused by trauma does not subside without treatment. Threats are seen everywhere.

In my altered perceptual state, I feel like a gladiator being sent to the lion's den to entertain a bloodthirsty audience. Below the level of consciousness, the "fight" in the flight or flight response to stress is reactivated.

When stress is at a minimum, the symptoms of STS abate. But as stress increases, or worse, becomes chronic, it can wreak havoc on the body resulting in anxiety, insomnia, muscle pain and a depletion of the immune system. Our bodies release hormones in response to normal stress to enable coping. But when the stress is long term, hormone release is prolonged, increasing the risk of illnesses such as cardiovascular disease. Feelings of helplessness and loss of control can lead to depression and suicidal thoughts.

Chapter 24

Despite caring for hundreds of patients and their families in my life, there have been very few I have disliked. Maria is definitely one of them. She has a way of getting under my skin like no other.

Maria is the primary caregiver for her aging mother. They recently moved into the geographical area I cover.

Early one Monday morning she calls. Before I can finish my greeting, Maria demands to receive homemaking assistance *"Right Away!"* Through her heavy accent, I am able to make out that Maria and her family care for her elderly mother because she is "sick, very, very sick." She goes on to explain that prior to the move, her mother was receiving home care on a daily basis.

"Daily?"

"Yes, yes nurse, because she is sick ... very, very sick."

With the recent budgetary cuts, daily home care is restricted to patients considered terminally ill. I wonder if Maria is struggling to find the correct English words for palliative care. Quickly I shuffle through my In Box, wondering if I had missed an urgent transfer request from the sending agency, but there is nothing.

"Maria, tell me about your mother's health."

Maria's voice raises several decibels. "*What?* Are you *stupid?* I told you already, she's *sick* ... very, very *sick!*"

I disregard her remark, knowing full well that in emergencies people often panic, say and do desperate things. I begin to wonder if I should call 911.

"Maria, is your mother breathing okay?"

Maria slowly draws in air through her nostrils, as if counting. I can sense her frustration with me. I am certain that she is rolling her eyes in disgust.

"She breathes fine, okay, but she's *worse.*" Her voice begins its ascent once again, "What do you *think?* No homemaker all weekend, boxes *everywhere.* Mess *everywhere. No wonder she's worse!*"

I pause to take in what she just said.

"So Maria, you're telling me that your mother is worse today because the house is messy?"

"*Fiii-nally,* you get it! Are all of you there so smart?"

Okay, my turn to take a deep breath. Anxiety, angst, negativity – all of it has a way of festering, and the last thing I need is to get caught up in the abyss of Maria's turmoil.

By this point several people in the office are glancing over with raised eyebrows, able to hear the muffled, high-pitched screeching coming from my receiver. I turn to face the corner of my cubicle.

"Well, are you sending someone now?" Maria asks.

I pause for another big breath. I doubt my response will be well received.

"I'm afraid I won't be able to send someone until after I make a home visit." It was our policy, and a reasonable one at that.

"So you're coming today, right?"

I glance at my appointment book; full day of appointments. The next few days are also completely booked.

"Well, I suppose I could come by at noon today."

Maria proves to be just as trying in person as she is on the phone. She greets me at the door of their brand new three-storey townhouse. I am led to the top level, up three steep staircases, to Maria's mother's room. An elderly woman waiting patiently, emanating a gentle demeanour, sits on the edge of a bed. A friendly, welcoming smile spreads across her face accentuating her delicate features and soft brown eyes. Her fragile hands dappled with age spots clasp the beads of a wooden rosary. I sit beside her and say hello.

Maria waves a hand in the air. "What do you know about her, she doesn't speak English. You need to talk to me."

"Can you tell your mother, I'm very pleased to meet her?" I place my hand over the woman's hand and smile. Maria speaks to her mother in their language. I begin to ask simple questions trying to determine what help this woman needs. By the end of an hour and a half, all I have really determined, beside the fact that she is "sick, very, very sick" is that at some time in the last year Maria's mother had a stroke that affected the left side of her body. Her leg drags slightly when she walks and her arm hangs limply, but she can still grasp items in her hand. She appears clean and neatly groomed. When I begin asking questions about the need for help with bathing, Maria appears confused.

"Can your mother wash herself? Does she need help with the bath?"

Maria waves her hand in the air again. "Yes, yes, she can do that, but she can't vacuum, can't clean."

"Well Maria, I'm afraid that our home care program, which likely runs a little differently from the one you're used to, can only allow a homemaker to visit if a person needs help with bathing."

Maria stands, at a temporary loss for words. Her eyes shift from left to right as she thinks about what I have said.

"No, *no!*" suddenly the words explode from Maria. "My English is not so good. She needs bath, sometimes very, very dirty." Maria begins waving the air around her backside. "Sometimes smelly, very, very smelly."

"Maria, where is the closest bathroom to your mother's room?"

Maria points down to the second floor.

"Wouldn't it be better if your mother was closer to the bathroom? And maybe close enough that she wouldn't have to go down a set of stairs?"

That question seems to rekindle her animosity. "What do you think, I don't know what's good for her? She has a nice room. She's up here, it's nice, it's quiet for her."

She's up here. I wonder about her life. How much time does she spend up here? What is their relationship like? I can't help but wonder about Maria's motives for keeping her mother in her home.

"Well Maria, I think there are several things we can do. We will send someone to help your mother bathe, but I will also send someone called an occupational therapist who will make sure your mother is safe to go up and down those stairs. She will see if you need any extra equipment in your home, things that will help your mother do more for herself.

"But the homemakers, when can they come?" It was becoming clearer by the minute that Maria had grown accustomed to having hired help in her home. By taking in her frail, elderly mother, I suspect Maria is reaping the benefits.

Over the next few weeks, my suspicions are confirmed when reports from the homemaking agency keep coming in with complaints of Maria's demands that homemakers complete the list of items on her "to do" list, none of which ever involve her mother. Then the occupational therapist's report arrives; Maria will only agree to those recommendations that are publicly funded. The suggestion to move her mother to a lower level, closer to a bathroom, is flatly refused. I am at a loss. Every gut instinct in me is saying that this woman is taking advantage of the system. I shudder to think what might happen if the benefits she reaped were no longer available.

In the course of the next year, I have frequent discussions with Maria, many having to do with her attempts at utilizing homemakers for her own personal use, not her mother's. Each time she is bad-tempered and eventually hangs up on me. I request reports from services going into the home looking for any signs of abuse. But there aren't any. Our relationship grows increasingly strained.

§§§

Caregiver burden refers to the strain experienced by "informal" caregivers such as spouses, family members or friends. The role can be very demanding. The caregiver's ability to cope is often dependant on factors such as the quality of the relationship with the person receiving the care, the degree of social isolation, and how well the caregiver understands the person's condition. As in any kind of stress, it is subjective. What one person might cope with, another might struggle with.

In home care, part of the assessment of any patient includes how well the caregiver is coping. At the time, I was convinced that Maria was only concerned about herself, and was using her mother's care as a means of getting publicly funded assistance for her own benefit. I still believe that was the case, but I can't help but wonder if cynicism – another side effect of STS – had a role in the dysfunctional relationship between Maria and me.

With the development of cynicism, you become easily irritated with patients; you are sure they are trying to drive you crazy. You can appear cold and uncaring. One of the key components of caring for the sick, and their families, is the ability to connect with them, and for them to recognize that connection. Cynicism is one of the effects of STS that extends beyond the individual, impacting others. Is it possible that I was discounting Maria's caregiver burden and minimizing her distress, and by so doing accentuating the strain on her?

Chapter 25

Sleep provides a temporary relief from the burden of my thoughts, but like mining for an elusive gem, not every attempt brings success. Most nights I toss in a tangle of covers and watch the clock as it reads 1:00, 2:00 then 3:00 a.m. Eventually exhausted, my mind gives in to much-needed sleep. But the moment I stir, even before my eyes open, I feel the familiar sense of dread run through me like a current seeping into each cell until every joint aches and every muscle hurts. I feel that I just can't go on.

With the funding cuts in the community sector of health care, the services I am able to provide my patients are significantly reduced. Guidelines for services are revised, and almost overnight I go from providing services to having to make drastic cuts. This doesn't sit well with me, and I teeter on the brink of a reality that threatens to loosen and give way. I have seen it before in the eyes of patients who are losing their minds. It doesn't matter what circumstances brings you to that edge, just that you are there and at risk of unravelling. I struggle to keep my thoughts rational, breathing my way through the panic of a racing heart and a throat that wants to clamp shut. I have gone from witnessing the suffering of others to inflicting it.

Can you imagine looking into the face of a ninety-three-year-old woman and having to tell her that she no longer qualifies for the help that she needs to remain in her own home? Because she doesn't fit the new criteria. That even though she had hoped she would never have to go to a nursing home, it now seemed inevitable? Patients dread my phone calls; they know what's going on. Many make excuses for appointment times, trying their best to postpone it, but for the most part they are housebound and run out of excuses before long. I call one woman who says she plans to have the local television network present during our visit. I think about how uncomfortable that will be, but tell her to do what she thinks best; it won't make a difference. When I arrive, the media is not present, and I am almost disappointed.

I schedule a visit with another woman who receives only a couple hours a week of homemaking help. I know the impact of my visit; it will significantly affect her ability to remain in her home. What little help we provide is enough to make the difference. The patient's daughter is present when I tell her mother that she will no longer get help with laundry. And since she doesn't receive help with a bath, she will be discharged from the program. The daughter argues that her mother requires that help. That family are not able to help out any more than they already are. I sit and nod, and say I am sorry. She walks me to the door as I am leaving.

"How can you look at yourself in the mirror?" Her voice almost a hiss.

"I can't," I tell her as I leave.

§§§

With secondary traumatic stress, it is not uncommon to shut down or cut yourself off from others. Subconsciously, in an attempt to block painful feelings, you can become desensitized to others. Emotionally overwhelmed, you find ways to keep out any additional distress. As a result, you may appear insensitive, as if you've "run out of compassion." This is a symptom of the silencing response referred to earlier.

During this time, there is no doubt many of my patients would have thought I was insensitive to their needs, even uncaring. And yet I felt every hurt I inflicted. My hands were tied. My job went from helping to hurting, and that didn't bode well for me. The only way I could navigate this experience was to tell myself that at least I was attempting to break the bad news to patients with as much compassion as possible. One of the most difficult things in life is when your values conflict with what you are expected to do at a job you depend on.

Chapter 26

I am helping the boys with their homework after dinner. Mike is struggling with math equations and Matt is working on colouring a map. The boys start arguing over an eraser, or a ruler, I'm not sure which. I start yelling. I swipe a book off the table, and it knocks over a plant. The dirt from the planter spreads across the floor. The boys look frightened. Bill is standing in the doorway, a look of concern mixed with frustration on his face. It's not the first time I've lost my cool.

"Leave. I'll take over."

I crawl into bed and close my eyes. The scene replays in my mind. *What's happening to me?*

I awaken before the sun comes up. It is Friday and I decide to call in sick and make an appointment to see my doctor. In his office, I tell him how tired I am. He is a young physician, astute enough to delve beyond the physical symptoms. He knows I work for the home care program and is well aware of the funding cuts. He immediately asks how things are going at work. He places my chart on his desk and swivels his chair around so that we are face to face. I tell him how difficult it is to carry out directives that I disagree with and how I went into nursing to help not harm. My voice cracks as I speak. His gaze is fixed and intent on me, and for the first time in a long time I feel that someone is really listening. He shakes his head in dismay and says, "That must be awful." Whether it is his understanding or a build-up of stored emotions, a river of tears breaks free and I struggle to collect myself.

"I'm sorry ... I don't know what's gotten into me," I say between sobs. "It's just ... well, it's just that it's so hard, you know? It doesn't sit well with me. I went into nursing thinking I'd be helping people. What I am doing is harming them." I babble on for much longer than my appointment time allows, grateful for his empathy.

He sends me home with a prescription for Ativan, a drug used for anxiety, and tells me to take a week off. The prescription is for five tablets. I take one pill that first night and sleep like I have never slept before. I understand why he only gave me five. Even I know how susceptible I am right now to pills that bring such sweet relief. A restful weekend and much-needed sleep make me feel that I can go on. I return to work on Monday. There are three pills left. I will carefully conserve them. Just knowing I have something to fall back on boosts my reserves.

§§§

When we are faced with prolonged stress, diminished self-care, moral distress and social isolation, an emotional breakdown is almost inevitable. I knew I was on the edge, and yet after my experience with the employee assistance counsellor, I was reluctant to seek help. There is a stigma attached to seeking mental health care, possibly more so for health care professionals who are used to helping, not being helped. The status quo is "suck it up and carry on." No one wants to be seen as someone who isn't coping.

Reflecting back now, it seems so clear. Self-compassion was absent. I had never heard of the term self-care. Fortunately, today the concept is well known. There are numerous articles, books and blogs on the need for self-care. It is a necessary component in both the prevention and the treatment of STS. Mother Teresa was well aware of this, insisting that the nuns in her convent take a one-year leave of absence every four or five years. We are all like wells that constantly need replenishing, and engaging in self-care activities helps to replenish the well. Self-care applies to everyone, but it is particularly important for people working in jobs that are emotionally demanding.

Chapter 27

A few months later, Bill receives a job offer from a company in Winnipeg. I know very little about the city but am willing to go anywhere just to be free of all the adversity I have experienced over the last few years. The negotiations can't happen fast enough for me. When the contract is sealed, I breathe a sigh of relief and hand in my resignation.

The large, old stone house we are living in has many outstanding renovations to be done before we can put it on the market. Even though I love the house and have told Bill on many occasions that I would be happy to die there, I am ready to move on.

Bill makes the move within a few weeks, flying home on weekends. The kids and I stay behind so I can oversee the last of the renovations. For over a year I have been refinishing the baseboards, doors and staircase. I finish up the woodwork while the tradesman update the upstairs bathroom and put new hardwood floors in the living room. The kids and I fly out to meet Bill one weekend and we go house hunting. By the end of the weekend we have purchased a house that is only two years old and requires no renovations. Although everything is chaotic, I couldn't be more pleased.

About ten days before the scheduled move, the kids are over at friends' homes and Bill and I are working on the house when we break for supper.

"Do you feel like going out?" Bill's clothes are splattered in paint.

"Hmmn, that would mean we have to get cleaned up. Besides, you have to eat out all week, you're probably sick of it. Why don't I just whip up something quick?"

"Are you sure? We could always order in."

"No, I'll just make Salisbury steak." I begin preparing our meal and go to open a can of vegetables. The can opener is finicky and only cuts through three quarters of the lid. In an attempt to pry it back, I cut my left index finger.

"Ow!" Blood starts oozing from it immediately and I rinse it under the tap. It feels like a deep cut. When I go to dry my hand I realize the finger will not bend. It is poker straight.

"What happened?" Bill heard my squeal and is at my side. "Do you think you need stitches?"

"I am afraid it might be more than that. I think I sliced the tendon."

We spend a couple of hours in the emergency department only to have my suspicions confirmed. I am referred to a specialist for surgical repair. In the whirlwind of our remaining days, I have surgery, attend physiotherapy and oversee the bulk of the packing. Added to my list of things to do is finding a physician in Winnipeg who is taking on new patients and who can refer me to a plastic surgeon for follow-up care.

On the day we leave, I turn the key in the lock for the last time and place a hand on the ornately carved wood door. There is so much about this house I love. Its beach stone wraparound porch, the large sprawling lawn, the in-ground pool we put in.

But so many of my memories are mired in malevolence. I turn to go, deciding that this move is going to be all about healing – body, mind and soul.

*

The saga of my left index finger drags on for months. It becomes obvious soon after the move that the distal joint repair did not take. I end up requiring two more surgeries to repair the tendons, leaving me with an index finger with limited movement. The chances of regaining full range of motion are slim. The severed area is referred to as "no man's land," difficult to repair. My recuperation time is spent thinking about what lies ahead career-wise.

On the night of my last surgery, as I am wheeled in from the recovery room, the nurse asks if I'd like something for pain. She whispers so as not to awaken my roommate. I nod, and when she returns, she assists me onto my side so I can swallow the pills. She helps me recline afterwards, checks the dressing on my finger, fusses with my pillows and places an extra blanket over me. Small and seemingly insignificant gestures that make all the difference. I drift off to sleep thinking, *Oh, she is so going to get chocolates from me.*

*

According to Eastern traditions, our bodies contain centres of energy called chakras that interact with various physiological and neurological systems within the body. There are seven main chakras positioned from the base of your spine to the crown of your head. It is believed that chakras help regulate all bodily processes including organ function, immune system and emotions. If a chakra becomes blocked, vital chi or prana is blocked and illness can occur.

I reach for my throat. *Could my throat chakra be blocked?* All the tests I have had show nothing, and yet the lump in my throat persists. I research further and learn about reiki, an energy healing treatment used to restore energy flow. Several weeks pass as I consider getting a reiki treatment. None of my friends have heard of it. Energy medicine is one of those complementary therapies that the medical field usually undermines because of a lack of scientific evidence proving its effectiveness. I decide to give it a try.

The reiki practitioner lives in an area of the city I rarely venture into, which pleases me. The chances of running into someone I know are small. Kara's credentials include a list of things I have never heard of: lightarian rays and shamanism. But she has extensive reiki training, and so I call her up and make an appointment.

When I arrive, Kara escorts me down to her treatment room, located on the lower level of her home. She sits on a couch and pats the cushion next to her. We spend the next half hour talking about what it is that has brought me to her. I tell her about my throat, about my curiosity if it might be blocked energy. She just nods, taking in all that I have to say. I ask about her "other" training, and she tells me it is part of her toolbox, so to speak, of things she uses to help her clients. Kara has a very endearing way about her. She is gentle, soft-spoken and exudes a calm that I have never before seen in anyone.

Next she has me lie down on a massage table that is centred in the room. I am covered in a blanket. Music plays softly and I hear the sounds of ocean waves.

I close my eyes and hear her standing above me, whispering. Briefly I open my eyes, but when I see she is not speaking to me, I close them again. I allow myself to relax, which is easy to do in the hands of someone I already trust. For the next hour I slip away into a deep state of relaxation, occasionally resurfacing when I become aware of her hands hovering over various parts of my body, or when her breathing changes from slow and rhythmic to several successive deep exhalations. Then all is quiet again.

I see Michael, my son. He is walking in a busy public area, maybe a mall. Two girls are with him, one blonde, the other brunette. I sense myself feeling on guard, not pleased with the situation.

Everything fades away. I am aware of Kara's breath on the exposed part of my arms.

Light puffs of air that make my hairs stand on end.

I see my other son, Matt. He is standing in front of a doorway and is about to enter when the door slams abruptly, leaving him stunned on the outside.

I open my eyes and Kara is sweeping her arms across my torso as if to brush away the air. Gently she places her hand on my arm and whispers, "Whenever you are ready."

We spend the next half hour talking about the session. I have more concerns now about the *dreams* I experienced than the reason I came. She explains to me that it is not uncommon to have visions during a session, nor is it uncommon to experience messages. She mentions something about meeting my spirit guide, but that information falls well beyond my level of understanding. I don't know how to respond, so I just nod politely. I leave, feeling mystified by the experience but really calm.

A few days later, I realize the sensation in my throat is gone. I take myself off the Nexium and my symptoms do not return.

A few weeks later, Michael introduces me to his "girlfriend." With them is her friend. One blonde, one brunette. I feel a great unease about entering a whole new phase of motherhood.

A few weeks after that, Matthew tries out for an AA hockey team, makes it through the first and second tryouts only to get cut in the third and final one.

§§§

Mainstream medicine is rooted in the idea that disease is a result of genetics and/or environment. In contrast, many of the alternative medical fields have long believed that disease is often a result of unresolved emotions and that thoughts and feelings can have an overwhelmingly significant impact on cells in the body. Thoughts are energy, and energy can become trapped. Emotions trigger the release of various chemicals: positive emotions like love and compassion release the "feel good" hormones. Emotional stress and anger trigger the release of cortisol, which can be useful in the short term but harmful in prolonged episodes. Blood sugar imbalances, suppressed immune system, decreased bone density, suppressed thyroid function and increased blood pressure are just a few of the possible negative effects.

Since there was nothing traditional medicine could do for my throat, I sought out alternative therapy. Not because I had lost faith in traditional medicine, but because I recognize that sometimes it is more than just our physical bodies that need healing.

Chapter 28

When my finger is healed, I decide it is time to get back to work. Like a moth to a flame, I decide to go back to bedside nursing. Whether I am trying to prove something to myself or trying to stay clear of previous experiences, I'm not sure. After updating my skills and knowledge of medications, I accept a position on a geriatric rehabilitation unit.

Late one evening, in the middle of my stretch of night shifts, my co-workers and I find ourselves struggling to keep up with patients' requests. Call bells are continuously ringing with requests for pain pills, sleeping pills, and assistance to the bathroom. Ann and Helen, the nurse and health care aide working along with me, joke light-heartedly that since it's not a full moon, it must be my vibrant crimson scrubs that are having a rousing effect on the patients.

To top things off, we have Bert to contend with. Bert is an emaciated, elderly man who suffers from dementia. Only Bert isn't the quiet, pleasantly confused type of dementia patient; he is prone to aggressive tendencies. Bert seems determined to spend his remaining days yelling obscenities and pitching anything within reach at anyone who might venture into his room.

Although he can get loud and disruptive, Bert's frail and feeble body doesn't pose much of a physical threat.

Around 2:00 a.m., I carefully peer into Bert's room. He is lying in his bed, covers strewn, rubbing his right ear.

"Get the hell out of here!" he yells. I pause for a moment, scanning the bedside table for objects that could potentially take flight, and then enter the room with caution.

"I said, get the hell out of here!"

"Bert, I see you're rubbing your ear. Is your head aching?" We all know that Bert rubs his ears when he is in pain.

"Yeah, damn headaches. But don't even try and give me any Tylenol. I'm not gonna take any Tylenol."

Bert eventually agrees to a warm drink. I help him to the side of the bed and sit with him as he slowly sips the warm milk. After a few minutes of light conversation, I sense that he is actually enjoying the company. As I sit there listening to Bert ramble on, I can't help but smile. *Yes, this is what I was missing.* When he finishes, I resettle him back into bed and tuck the covers close by his unshaven face. He closes his eyes and in minutes falls into a deep and restful sleep.

The next night, when I peer into Bert's room, he is haphazardly making his way from the bathroom.

"How's everything tonight, Bert?"

Bert straightens slowly to acknowledge me, and then glances at me from head to toe.

"Shit," he mutters. "I was hoping it was that lady in red."

Before long, the dreams are back. I drive to work praying for an easy day, no emergencies, no palliative care patients. I drive home thinking about all the things I might have forgotten. Things begin to spiral, I no longer see things objectively, reading far more into things than I should. It's as if I am in some hyper-alert state, always seeing the worst that could happen. It becomes draining and once again I drag myself into work every day exhausted, confused and at a loss as to what is going on.

*

I am hurrying the boys out the door, hoping they haven't missed the school bus, when the phone rings. It's my good friend, Danita. Her voice sounds strained and I ask her if everything's okay.

"Dorothy, it's my dad. His cancer is back."

I sit down, the words already running a chill down my spine. The faces of patients I have cared for flash before me, people whose lives were turned upside down by a disease that eventually robbed them of life. Twenty-some odd years come barrelling into the moment.

Aware that I haven't said anything, I struggle to find words of comfort, hoping not to hear that he is palliative, but nothing comes to me.

"The doctor says he doesn't have long."

She is sobbing softly, and my heart is breaking for her. "Oh Danita, I am so sorry."

"I'm going to fly out tomorrow, to be with him. He wants to stay at home as long as he can."

"Yeah, that's a good idea. Is there anything I can do? You'll call me, won't you, if you need anything?"

Danita and I have been friends for years. We were introduced at our husbands' employee Christmas party in December '97. While our children took part in the organized games and our husbands were off discussing work, we sat at the back of the large auditorium, beneath streamers of shiny tinsel and speakers piping out songs about jolly old St. Nick. Danita was warm and friendly, and made me feel at ease. We formed an instant connection.

As the years go by, our friendship becomes less about our husbands' careers and more about us. On many fronts we are different. She grew up a devoted Zionist; I was raised Catholic. After high school, Danita spent some time living in a kibbutz in Israel. For spring break, I headed to Daytona Beach. Even our children are vastly different. While her kids are touring human rights museums, mine are tearing up tracks on their dirt bikes in the vacant field out back. Our differences add to the diversity of our friendship. We meet regularly for lunches and talk about everything from books and parenting to spirituality and the meaning of life. We have been through a lot together, including a major cross-country move, one that would have been daunting had we not had each other.

I hang up the phone, at a loss as to what to do. What can I do? What can anyone do? I rub my hands together trying to get some warmth into them. My breakfast is tumbling in my belly like a ball in a bingo cage. My heart is racing and I have to remind myself to take deeper breaths. It's like I've just run a marathon.

I head to the bedroom to get a sweater, but by the time I reach the room I am gripped with terror. I need to lie down. I pull back the covers and crawl inside. Don't think about it. There is nothing you can do right now. But what if she needs advice on home care or pain meds, or any number of things I can't fathom at the moment? Tomorrow, you can call her tomorrow.

Warmth begins to seep back, first into my hands, and then my feet.

A few days go by and with it comes the gnawing ache of knowing I haven't called her yet. But every time I go to pick up the phone, the sensations return: my hands then feet get cold, there's a loud thumping in my chest, and I am terrified. I tell myself she knows how to reach me, she'll call if she needs me. I convince myself that if I call I'll probably be interrupting something important like a visit from the doctor. She won't be able to talk anyway.

Two weeks go by and I still don't pick up the phone. Every day I wrestle with a guilt that wraps around my neck like a scarf tied too tight. Each night I ask myself what kind of friend am I? If our situations were reversed, she'd be in constant contact. But I just can't pick up the phone. It's not procrastination that's stopping me, it's inability. The thought of calling paralyses me. My body and mind aren't willing to do what my heart is directing it to do. I can't bear to face her situation.

A few days later, the phone rings. It's my husband calling from work.

"Dorothy, Danita's dad died last night."

I sink into a chair. I want to scream. My hands cover my face.

"Dorothy, are you there?"

After a few moments I answer. "Yeah, I'm here."

"Are you okay?" Bill seems puzzled. He gets that I am sad for Danita, but probably wonders why I'm taking it so hard since I never met her father.

He has no idea how angry I am with myself, that I am chastising myself for not reaching out to a friend when she needed me most. Every day I made excuses. Not because I don't care, but because it hurts too much to care. Who have I become? Will Danita ever be able to forgive me? Will I ever be able to forgive myself?

§§§

This incident was my wake-up call. I knew I could no longer blame stress or burnout; something much more insidious was going on. I would continue to nurse for another year, and in that time recognize that my perception and judgment – crucial skills in health care – were impaired. I would begin to see that I was no longer the person I used to be, someone who loved the company of family and friends and saw joy in simple moments. Instead, I lived as if tragedy lurked around every corner. My impaired skills would eventually lead to my resignation, at the age of forty-five.

Part 3
2006–2014

The best way out is through.
—Robert Frost

Chapter 29

I pick up the photo of the soldier, seeing things differently now. I'll never know how his story ended, but I know I have a choice as to how mine will. Secondary Traumatic Stress does not have to be a life sentence, and I am determined to do whatever I can to ensure it isn't. Although I can't unwind the clock to erase my experiences, there are many things I can do to begin healing. Learning as much as I can about STS seems like the most logical place to start. In my search for information, I come across Green Cross Academy of Traumatology and see that they offer a course on assessment and treatment of STS in Minnesota, about an eight-hour drive from my home. I immediately sign up.

Dr. Chase greets our small group in the meeting room of an AmericInn Hotel. I collect my handouts and glance at the other students, wondering about their backgrounds. No one acknowledges me or anyone else, preferring to glance through the handouts or ready their workspace. It feels a little impersonal. Of the many courses and workshops I've attended over the years, in the few minutes before sessions start, I have always engaged in some interaction with fellow students even if it was as simple as a smile and an introduction. But not this time.

Each person seems to have drawn an imaginary box around himself or herself that defines where personal space begins and ends. I scan the room and see that everyone is scattered spaciously apart. There are only a handful of us. I find a chair in a vacated area to the far left. I'm guessing there won't be a pool party tonight.

Dr. Chase begins by suggesting that we introduce ourselves and explain a little about why we are here. As each person stands, I am amazed at how diverse a group we are. Among us are a volunteer firefighter, a clerk for a social service agency, a vet and an early childhood educator. There are no health care-related professionals other than myself. Although it saddens me, it doesn't surprise me. Health care has been slow to recognize the damaging effects of STS.

Over the course of the next two days, Dr. Chase goes into detail about the effects of STS, its root cause, the symptoms and treatment modalities. We learn about the body's response to STS, the structural changes that occur in the brain. Since the brain is neuroplastic, it can change again. Circuitry can be rewired. The participants share experiences and, in doing so, warm to one another. By the end of the workshop, each of us feels equipped to speak about something that previously we had no language for. We say our goodbyes and thank Dr. Chase, and I return to my hotel room, certificate in hand, feeling hopeful.

As I glance through the material, I can't help but think about the nursing profession. Nursing shortages are becoming a global concern. Equally problematic are the turnover and exit rates of RNs. Since nurses are the largest group of professionals within the global health care system, these exit rates will have a huge impact on health care as we know it. So many of the studies of nurses who leave the profession early cite emotional exhaustion

– a symptom of STS – as one of the reasons. I think back to when I left, and my inability to articulate why.

Not unlike the past when little was known about PTSD, it is time to stop ignoring the issue of STS and to recognize the full impact it can have. In a field where human suffering and heartache is witnessed daily, it's time to ensure that everyone is equipped with the necessary knowledge of what STS is and how it can affect people. It's time to consider providing support such as debriefing in workplaces and employee assistance programs capable of treating STS with counselling and EMDR (eye movement desensitization reprocessing). It's time to impart knowledge about STS at the ground level of training for careers. But most important of all, it's time that STS is no longer dismissed as something only the weak develop. It can happen to anyone.

Chapter 30

As part of my healing process, I decide to try EMDR. Eye movement desensitization reprocessing is a recommended treatment for STS. It works primarily with the disturbing memories. I spend some time perusing websites of psychologists and find a few that list *traumas* as a specialty. The website for Dr. Rushton has a photograph of him, a list of his specialties and a few key questions. "Missing out on the best of life? Not living up to your potential? Ready to move past obstacles?" I feel that he already knows me.

Initially we correspond by email. I tell him upfront that I suspect I am suffering from STS and want to see if EMDR will help. All I really know about this technique is that research on its effectiveness sounds promising. We arrange an appointment to meet.

I sit alone in the waiting room of the office that Dr. Rushton shares with a few other practitioners. I am grateful that even if someone else does come in, they won't know whether I am waiting for a massage, a counsellor or a homeopathic doctor. That thought nags at me; I would not think little of anyone else seeking therapy, so why do I feel embarrassed that I need help? I look up at the receptionist who is busy with paperwork.

How many people in a day does she see who come in looking as sheepish as me? My thoughts are interrupted when Dr. Rushton appears in the waiting room. He greets me warmly with an outstretched arm. I follow him down the hall to his office, a tastefully decorated, dimly lit room. I sit on the couch across from his computer chair, and he swivels away from his desk to face me.

Dr. Rushton wastes no time in superficial niceties and dives directly into the heart of why I am there. We spend the next hour talking about my reasons for believing I have STS, about my career as a nurse and the residual effects I continue to have. At some point during the session, I know I've made the right choice in a therapist. As I describe things, like the panic I feel at the sound of a siren or the sense of paralysis when faced with the prospect of helping someone through an illness, Dr. Rushton listens in a caring and nonjudgmental way. I feel validated. For the first time in a long while, I feel that what I am saying is not being diminished or brushed aside. Then I realize the only person doing that was me. At the end of our session, I agree to meet him again in a week. I am to bring a list of memories I consider "critical moments."

Making the list is easy. I reach for the memories that have a way of triggering a whole set of physiological symptoms. Memories that make my heart race, my palms sweat, my breaths short. First on my list is Daniel, the seventeen-year-old victim of a motor vehicle accident. Swirling around those painful memories is the intensity of grief I experienced with his mother. In no time, I have listed eight critical moments.

Our next session begins with a brief discussion about EMDR.

"You are going to follow my fingers as you think over the details of this memory."

"Follow your fingers?" It is not what I expected, maybe something that involves electrodes and equipment.

"I will be moving my hand back and forth. Keep your eyes focused on my fingers at all times."

I nod, wondering how in the world this will make any difference. But I have enough trust in Dr. Rushton to give it a try. Keeping my eyes on his fingers, I think back to that night so long ago. My senses prickle with the adrenalin rush of being called to emerg. The limp and lifeless body of a seventeen-year-old wheeled in. The flap of his scalp, his jet black hair, the trickle of blood on his face. I can feel a panic rise within. A sort of pleading with God, not to take him. He's too young. I continue to follow Dr. Rushton's fingers. I can smell the dampness of Daniel's blood-soaked clothing as the attendants take hold of the back board and, in one swift motion, transfer him onto the trauma room stretcher. We descend on him in a flurry of activity, inserting IVs, hooking up a cardiac monitor, inserting an endotracheal tube, pumping the laeradal bag and resuming compressions on his chest. Dr. Rushton's fingers continue to glide from left to right. I see her. The mother. She is helpless. Barely conscious herself, she thinks only of her son and tries to reach for him. Her eyes glance at mine. Our gaze locks and I am filled with a horrific sense of grief. This moment goes on forever, me pumping vital air into his lungs, watching a mother lose her son. The monitor continues to show a cold flat line. I can barely see Dr. Rushton's fingers through the tears that have filled my eyes. He stops.

I wipe the tears with a tissue he gives me and blow my nose. We talk about the experience. The questions he asks and the way he rephrases things tell me he understands. With him there is no need to suck it up, to minimize the hurt.

"Shall we try it again?"

We start over. I follow his fingers. I go through the memory, through each of the details, saddened by it but feeling slightly different. The feelings surrounding this memory no longer feel all consuming. The intense panic is gone, and there is less of an emotional sting. Nothing changes the fact that Daniel died, but the gnawing is gone. It is like turning down the volume. The memory has become more bearable. All that with the movement of his fingers.

I leave that session in awe. I check myself throughout the rest of the day to see if the intensity returns, but it doesn't. I feel okay. But mostly I feel hopeful that EMDR will help put to rest the many unresolved emotional memories that have been eating away at me, bit by bit.

I meet with Dr. Rushton for a few more sessions of EMDR. I am in awe at how it works. Besides minimizing the intensity of emotion surrounding the memory, in a few cases I am able to see things this time around that I didn't see before, as if my perception has been cloudy. I wonder how many years I have been stumbling around without clarity of vision.

At our last session, I thank him, at a loss for words about how I really feel. For years, I knew something was wrong. For years, I watched information on STS grow and slowly disseminate, and yet still its importance among health care workers was dismissed.

Today, treatment of secondary traumatic stress and PTSD include EMDR, cognitive behavioural therapy and a program known as the Accelerated Recovery Program (ART). It is a five-session intensive training program for professionals suffering from the effects of STS. The aim of the program is to help resolve the symptoms and the cause of STS, as well as enhance future resiliency. I can't help but hope the program will find its way into the curriculum of medical, nursing and social work programs.

Chapter 31

Since much has been written about the holistic benefits of massage therapy, I begin regular sessions. As the therapist is kneading the knots out of my muscles, she comments that my spine is out of alignment and that I would benefit by a visit to the chiropractor, preferably one trained in Network Spinal Analysis (NSA). Although I have seen chiropractors over the years, this specialty is new to me. She goes on to explain it as a form of healing meant to achieve not only spinal wellness but of the nervous system as well.

"Stress has a way of accumulating in the body," she adds as she touches an area on my neck that always feels stiff and sore. "As a defence, the body locks these stressors into deep-rooted tension patterns. The precise, low force touches used in NSA has a way of unlocking these tension patterns, and assists you in becoming more in tune with your body."

I decide to read up on it and learn that so much of the focus of NSA is on the nervous system. Trauma can wreak havoc on the nervous system. According to the Network Chiropractors Canada website, NSA can provide benefits such as improvement in handling stress, decreased anxiety, greater flexibility of the spine and an improved awareness of your body. All things I need. I decide to give it a try.

Dr. Kish spends close to an hour on my initial assessment. A lot of questions are geared toward physical, chemical and emotional traumas. He assesses my spine for structural and facilitated subluxations that can create pressure on the nervous system. Finally, he has me lay on the table and applies precise touches to various areas on my neck and back in intervals. The relaxing music in the background lulls me into a deep state of calm. I occasionally sense my breath change, as if tension is being released.

With each visit I marvel at Dr. Kish's ability to know specifically what part of my back to treat. It is as if he knows where the tension is trapped. All I know is that within a few visits, I feel more limber, more hopeful, more in tune to my body. I decide NSA will remain part of my maintenance regime going forward.

*

Feeling more like myself than I have in years, I decide my next step is to take a really good look at self-care.

Self-care is recognized as an important ingredient in building resistance against STS. It is also crucial in healing from it. Health care professionals can easily fall prey to the philosophy that others' needs come first. It's an expectation during training as well as on the job. Couple that with life circumstances that keep you so busy that you have little time for yourself and it's easy to see how self-care can fall by the wayside. But I am reminded of my fortune cookie. *If you make yourself a mouse, you raise the possibility of being eaten by a cat.* There is no need to become a victim.

Whether it is caring for others or ourselves, so much of our ability to do so stems from our childhood and what we witnessed first-hand from parents. My mother epitomizes selflessness. I have a vivid memory of her in the kitchen, peeling potatoes for supper. She had just gotten home from work and was still wearing her coat. My mother did not take the time to meet her own needs before she was hurrying to meet ours. It was the way she cared for her family. Self-sacrificing behaviours are second nature to her.

On one occasion in my early adulthood, my mother and I visited a distant relative named Stella. The topic of conversation fell to parenting. Stella told us that before she tended to the needs of anyone else, she looked after herself. She got up every morning, bathed, dressed and got herself ready for the day, often eating breakfast before she thought about anyone else's needs. Her children knew not to make any requests of her until she was ready. We were surprised by this foreign concept. Equally surprising to us at the time was the pride in her words.

We drove home stunned by Stella's admittance. That was not how I was brought up, and consequently not the way I would eventually parent my children. But as the meaning of her words settled over us, I sensed their wisdom. Later I would learn that even the Dalai Lama, considered the guru of compassion, advises that if you want to help people, help yourself first. Self-care is a delicate balance between selflessness and selfishness.

I decide to make a list of self-care strategies. Taking the time for enjoyable hobbies, listening to music or reading a book, taking a bubble bath – these seemingly insignificant behaviours can make a difference. Connecting with nature, catching a nap or having lunch with a friend can help incorporate much needed "me" time. Self-care is a necessity, not a luxury.

Self-care at its very essence is self-compassion. For me, that will mean silencing my inner critic and practicing simple acts of kindness like focusing on things I like about myself or achievements I am proud of. I vow to smile more, even if it's just a *faux* smile, because stretching the facial muscles in that way triggers the brain to produce more endorphins. I decide I will make a conscious effort to notice positive feelings and experience the flood of "feel good" hormones.

Self-care includes nurturing your body by eating well, getting regular exercise and adequate rest. I already practice yoga, but not regularly enough. I will try meditation for relaxation and the release of negative emotions. I bump up the time I spend at the gym enrolling in classes that combine strength and cardio. By the time I am done thinking about self-care, I have made an impressively long list of things to do. Some of the self-care activities address the body, some the mind. Many include activities that excite me. Making a list of self-care activities is highly subjective. It needs to be based on individual preferences and interests.

Chapter 32

First on my list of self-care strategies is a much needed vacation. Ever since the kayaking trip, I have longed for another "me time" vacation. Since Bill has never been interested in taking a cruise, I decide it will be perfect. I plan to travel alone because I want to do whatever I feel like doing whenever, and a cruise seems like a safe place for a solo female traveller. In no time, I have the trip booked and can barely contain my excitement.

As I stand on the pier waiting to embark the *Caribbean Princess*, I can't believe the size of the ship. It is huge at almost 200 feet tall and almost 1,000 feet long. I'm not sure what to expect about the embarkation process and suspect that with more than 3,000 passengers to check in, I'll experience a wait but am surprised at how streamlined and efficient the lines are. In no time, I am leaving behind the clerk with my trusty ship map in hand and a promise that my luggage will be delivered to my room soon.

I make my way to the Aloha Deck to find my room. It's compact but pleasant. On the bed is a swan made of hand towels and a note from my room attendant encouraging me to call him if there is anything I need. On the desk is a bottle of wine, courtesy of my travel agent. I uncork the bottle, pour myself a glass and open the doors to my veranda. The salty smell of the ocean greets me. From here I take in the view of the pier and the skyline of Fort Lauderdale. I am hoping no one can see me because I am sure I am sporting the silliest of grins. I let out a big sigh. This week is going to be all about "me." Earlier this morning while waiting for the shuttle to the pier, I struck up a conversation with a couple who was also cruising. It was their third cruise, and they were happy to fill me in on what to expect: the food, the activities, the service. "Your attendant will make up the room in the morning and will return in early evening to turn down your sheets and leave chocolates on the pillow." I expressed uneasiness with that much attention, but they assured me I would grow to love it.

Also on the desk is the *Princess Patter,* the ship's newsletter listing each of the events going on for the day. I decide to take a guided tour of the ship so I'll have an idea where everything is located. It is so large it is like a city, with boutiques, five pools, numerous restaurants and bars and entertainment theatres. By the end of the tour, I am confident I can find my way to the buffet restaurant, the pool and my room. I am set.

The *Princess Patter* is delivered each evening, and I scrutinize it to plan my activities for the next day. Even on the days we are at sea, I rise early since there is so much to pack into seven days. With various arts and craft workshops like scrapbooking and ceramics, seminars on digital photography made easy, hypnosis, and eat more to weigh less, I am scrambling to get to everything I want to attend. The days at port are spent meandering around St. Marten and St. Thomas taking in the sights, the sounds and the shopping. At each port, I take an excursion that includes a tour of the island.

By the time the week draws to an end, I wish I had booked a ten or even a fourteen-day cruise. Although I cherish vacations with my family, this has been a vacation of a lifetime. I vow that from here on in, one week, maybe even two, each year will be just for me.

Chapter 33

Doodles. Sometimes bold geometric shapes, other times squirrely lines that dance across the page. As soon as the ink makes contact with the blank white page it seems to have a will of its own as pages fill with designs. Doesn't matter if it's lopsided, or one shape keeps repeating itself over and over; the expectation isn't to produce artwork. Whatever is inside is free to leave, liberated to the light of day. I feel like a bystander, watching over my shoulder as the contours spill out until little white space is left. That's when I get to work filling in the blanks with cerulean blues, neon pinks, orange as vibrant as an early morning sun. I am drawn to vibrant colours so the darker hues like brown, navy and forest green are seldom used, reserved for the darkest of moods.

Colouring was a favourite pastime when my kids were young. But my doodles predate that; they stretch back into my own childhood. I have been "colouring" forever. When my kids were small I quickly realized the calming effect it had on them. When Matt was hospitalized for an appendectomy, a box of crayons and blank paper went with me as I sat vigil by his bedside. Feeling so unwell, I couldn't convince him to pick up a crayon, but he wanted to watch me. The effect on him was tangible, his eyes glued first to my marker as I made my outline, and then to my hand and the melodic rhythm of colouring it in.

Much has been written on the benefits of art therapy. According to a literature review done by Stuckey and Nobel,[13] engaging in creative expression such as music therapy, dance, journaling and art can restore emotional balance, calm neural activity in the brain, help restore immune functioning and improve overall sense of well-being. Viktor Frankl, author of *Man's Search for Meaning*, believes our need to find meaning and relevance in our daily experiences is what drives artistic creation. It is an exploration, reflection and expression of what is going on inside, often on an unconscious level. Whether it's dance, poetry or painting, something happens when we engage in the arts regardless of our culture, age or health status. It is therapeutic.

As I colour in the last few shapes, I notice my page is filled with neon bright images that have an uplifting feel. I step back and view my work. At first glance it seems to be a chaos of shapes and colour. But then shapes begin to have form. There is stability in the geometric squares and rectangles. A conflict or tension in the triangles that sit tilted off their base. Amid the swirl of spirals is a feeling of motion and change. I can see wings, rays of sunshine and a question mark. I take a black marker and at the bottom of the page write, *If I let you in, will you like what you see?*

*

In an old briefcase, in a box in the basement, is my stash of journals. Years' worth of pouring out thoughts on paper, these journals chronicle good times and bad. Some date as far back as the late seventies, when I was in my teens. Throughout my life, journaling has always been a way to sort out feelings, record important events, explore solutions to problems and reflect on my life and what I was experiencing in that moment. It is an excellent tool for self-discovery. In an article titled, "Finding the Words to Say It: The Healing Power of Poetry," Robert Carroll writes:

> Our voices are saturated with who we are, embodied in the rhythms, tonal variations, associations, images and other somato-sensory metaphors in addition to the content of meaning of the words. Our voices are embodiments of ourselves, whether written or spoken. It is in times of extremity that we long to find words or hear another human voice letting us know we are not alone.[14]

Like poetry, journaling is a release. The words on the page are simply a way to process thoughts and feelings. In a journal, I allow myself to be completely truthful, free from criticism or judgment. Sometimes I write from an alternate perspective to try to see things from a different angle. Doing so allows some distance from myself and my thoughts, and often adds clarity. It can take an overwhelming feeling and replace it with curiosity. If I have difficulty getting started, feeling at a loss as to where to begin, I focus on one word. What I think may be at the core. *Scared. Withdrawn. Scattered.* Then I make bubbles around those words and fill them in with more sensations that randomly come to mind. *Worried. Alone. Confused.* Getting emotions onto the page is a process. Sometimes you have to dig deep. Inevitably, all roads lead home, and to the heart of the matter. My journals are not written for anyone else's eyes. One day I will burn them all, but for now I can't let go of them. They are an integral part of who I am and where I'm headed and how I heal.

I have a friend who uses a journal not to write in, but to express herself in visual imagery. She pastes pictures from old magazines that tell her story. She might add small items that can be easily glued in. Any text is added in with a gold coloured marker.

I used to carefully choose the journals I bought. They had a design that struck me as beautiful or intricate patterns embossed on the cover. But then I would hesitate to write in them, feeling that only well thought out verse was worthy of going in them. Now I choose plain composition books and write whatever needs to come out at the time.

Whether you write, draw or collage in a journal, it is all about release. It is a valuable tool for reflection, which is often the way we learn life's biggest lessons. It helps to organize thoughts, seek bigger meanings, explore new perspectives. It is a valuable tool in maintaining a sense of well-being.

*

Since gardening for so many is akin to therapy, I decide to plant a vegetable garden. Dreams of being self-sufficient with the cold storage room in the basement filled with an assortment of preserves and canned goods seem so enticing. I plan out the vegetable plot, being careful to place certain vegetables next to each other to optimize produce. I weed the garden plot and till the soil until I am satisfied my seedlings will be given the best start at life. I buy some vegetables, like tomatoes and squash, at my local nursery, and plant peas, carrots and corn from seeds. Every few days I water my garden, and weed again. Late spring turns into early summer and the mosquitoes arrive. At first I swat at the pesky creatures, then I spray repellent and wear long sleeves. Eventually those unrelenting bugs have me fleeing inside where I peer through my kitchen window at my vegetables.

Next come the rabbits and deer. All the kale and lettuce are gone, providing sustenance for them instead of us. I vow to build a critter-proof fence next year.

By the end of the season, the corn cobs are filled with tiny white worms, the potatoes are the size of golf balls, and there is no sign of cabbage amid their huge leaves.

Instead of my family reaping the harvest of my garden, I head to the local farmers' market where produce is plentiful. I drive home thinking about the hours I put into my garden and how little I received. I think back to the lush gardens of my childhood, picking peas off by the handful and eating them right out of their shells. All I have to show for my efforts are a few misshapen tomatoes and a handful of carrots. Although gardening may be a source of relaxation and nourishment for some, it is not for me. But finding self-care activities means trying out new things as well as tried and true ones.

Chapter 34

I knew things were turning around when the urge to volunteer returned. Volunteering is an opportunity to give your time, energy or skills to part of the community. Many volunteers expect little or nothing in return, and yet there are benefits to be reaped. Studies indicate that volunteering can be good for your health. Those who volunteer are said to have lower mortality rates and depression and greater functional ability than those who do not. Volunteering is a way to gain new skills, connect with others and help to improve lives. I scan through the list of opportunities on the web: clerical work for social service agencies, assistance with literacy programs, various charity events and a need for shut-in visitors. The last one interests me, but I wonder if I am ready. Will I be able to face the difficulties so often experienced with the elderly? Will I feel as if I am right back at home care? I decide I'll never know unless I try.

Rose is eighty-six years old and lives alone in a seniors' apartment. She has never been married and has no children. Although the complex has a meal plan and dining room, Rose prefers to stay in her own apartment and cook light meals in her small but functional kitchen. When I call to arrange a visit, Rose seems skeptical about why I am visiting. I can't help but be reminded of my days as a case manager when my visits were not welcomed. It is different this time, I tell myself.

When I arrive for my first visit, Rose needs reminding about who I am and why I am here. I describe again the shut-in visitors program that she herself had signed up for and review a list of things we can do when I come by. Although disappointed I'm not going to take her to the mall for shopping excursions, she is pleased with the idea of being read to. In the last few months, Rose's eyesight has been steadily failing. She can watch television but prefers to listen to the radio.

I suggest an old classic like something by Jane Austin or Louisa May Alcott, and we decide on *Emma*. Since I haven't brought any books for our initial meeting, we spend the rest of our time getting to know each other.

In the next few months, I visit Rose for an hour or two each week. During that time, I watch her progressively fail. At first, I try not to notice. I am not visiting her as a nurse. But then the risks of not speaking up become too apparent. I call the volunteer coordinator to share my concerns. She will speak to Rose's next of kin, a niece whom Rose has never mentioned.

A week later when I call Rose to arrange our visit, there is no answer. I call the staff at the seniors' apartment hoping she hasn't fallen and can't reach the phone. I am told that Rose was sent to a nursing home. I take note of where she went.

The doors to the nursing home are locked, with instructions to buzz the ringer for admittance. The door clicks and when I open it, a faint waft of urine accosts me. I head to the receptionist's desk to ask where I might find Rose. I am given a room number and shown which wing to take.

I find Rose sitting in a chair staring out a window that overlooks a small courtyard. Rose doesn't recognize me until I reintroduce myself. She looks as if she has aged ten years.

"It's not so bad here," Rose offers as if reading my concern for her. "They even serve tea and cookies in the evening." I reach over and take her hand.

"But it's nothing like home, so I am hoping I will get better soon and be able to go."

My hope of her acceptance drops a notch. I feel her inner turmoil; I know what she is going through. But I realize what is happening to me. I close my eyes briefly, wondering how I can stop myself from becoming a sponge. I focus on my breath for a few minutes, and when I do, something comes to me. *Don't focus on the outcome. Focus on the here and now.*

I open my eyes to find Rose watching me. I smile at her. If I can just focus on why I am here I might be able to recognize her hardship but not internalize it. I pull out the book and ask if she remembers where we left off. For now, and each time I visit with her, I will not think of Rose's predicament. I will think of our time together.

When I was in nursing school, we learned very little about boundaries. We were advised to avoid situations that might compromise nurse/patient relationships, such as getting intimately or sexually involved.

But there is so much more to boundaries than that. How we handle boundaries affects how open we are to experiencing another's suffering. Developing boundaries is a skill, an intricate balance that allows for empathy but doesn't overwhelm. But how exactly is that done? If we put up boundaries, doesn't that suggest closing ourselves off to compassion? When I spoke of this conundrum to a friend of mine who is a trained therapist, she explained boundaries in a much more palatable way. She suggested thinking about a boundary as something you have built – not a concrete wall, but a picket fence with slats wide enough to allow the information you need to know to filter in without it becoming too much. And that picket fence has a gate with a latch on the inside. You control when the door swings open.

This analogy hit home for me. I only wish I had learned it many years ago. It's at the crux of STS, when we either shut empathy down or let it cripple us. Finding a way to handle the powerful emotion of empathy is something all health care providers need to do for themselves and their patients.

Chapter 35

As part of my decision to fill my life with rich and engaging activities, I begin taking week-long courses every summer. I become intrigued by a workshop called Writer as Shaman. The syllabus describes it as a writing retreat that incorporates some shamanic teachings as a way to nurture your craft and your soul. I know very little about shamanism other than it is a type of spiritualism. Since mysticism and spirituality have always fascinated me, I decide to sign up. After I do, I read up on it and discover that a shaman is someone who perceives and interacts with the spirit world in order to channel certain energies and insights to this world. They often do so by reaching altered states of consciousness. This leaves me feeling uncertain, but each time I read the syllabus I get a surge of excitement: I have to go. I have no idea what to expect other than it is offered at the Cloquet Forestry Center, a beautiful retreat centre nestled in a forest of large white pines. I have always admired white pines; their windswept appearance reminds me that adversity can be overcome. I take this as a good omen.

Lying on my blanket on the classroom floor, I look around. Fellow participants are scattered around the room in various positions. Some on their backs, a few curled up in fetal position, whatever is comfortable the instructor has told us as she prepares us for our first journey. I am close to the exit, not by accident; I still have reservations about being here.

Our instructor, Ruth, begins by explaining that she teaches Core Shamanism, a program founded by Michael Harner. This type of shamanism integrates core beliefs from varying cultures. "A shaman is a person who interfaces with the spirit world," she tells us matter-of-factly, as if she is teaching us the fundamentals of geometry or geography. "We will be journeying into the lower world to meet our spirit guides. Shamans believe there are three worlds: upper, middle and lower. In the upper and lower worlds, only compassionate beings exist. We live in the physical portion of the middle world. But there is also the unseen part of the physical world, where entities such as ghosts exist." Her voice is calm and reassuring. She has a presence like no one I have ever met. She exudes a quiet confidence that has me trusting her enough not to pack my bags and head for home.

Ruth goes on to explain how journeying is giving yourself permission to have awakening dreams. At any point, you can choose to end a journey. If you find yourself believing that you are making it all up, simply trust that the images that come to mind are for a purpose. Journey with intention; go with a specific question, a desire for direction or guidance. Everyone has the ability to access other realms. And everyone has spirit guides.

Ruth finishes off by performing a smudging ritual; an abalone shell holds the burning embers of sage leaves. With a large feather, she fans the embers of this sacred plant so that tiny wisps of smoke spread through the room. The sweet earthy scent tickles my nostrils. She places the vessel down and picks up a drum. Slowly and rhythmically she begins to beat the drum.

I take a deep breath and close my eyes. I feel the twitching of muscles, and then relaxation. She begins to lead us through our first journey.

I leave my cottage shoreline and head by kayak to an island I know has a deep crevice in the face of a rock. I slide the kayak into the crevice, feeling sheltered and cradled on three sides by the rock. The waves lap gently against the kayak and I sink deeper into myself, so deep that I feel like I have sunk into my stomach. It is dark there and I call out for my spirit guide. Nothing.

I get up and walk deeper into the cave, feeling uneasy. A beam of light appears and I walk toward it. The cave opens up to the top of a hillside, and once again I call for my spirit guide. Suddenly a vision of a bald eagle flashes through my mind. Did I make that up? I call out to the eagle to come, but it circles high in the sky, wings outstretched, a silhouette against the setting sun. Just when I think it is flying away, it changes direction and lands not far from where I am standing. I blurt out a series of questions. "Are you my spirit guide? What do I need? Why am I here?" I pause. Nothing. I wait. I get an overwhelming feeling that all I need to do right now is sit in the eagle's presence. I am okay with that because I also get a strange reassuring feeling that my questions will get answered in time. But for now I just need to be still.

"Be still and know I am here."

The words are loud and audible. Those words are biblical, and I feel reassured that none of this is against my traditional Christian beliefs. Many paths up the mountain. At this point, the drumming changes. Ruth is calling us back. I return the way that I came, back through the cave to the kayak and then to the shoreline of my cottage.

A few days into the workshop we are encouraged to go outside and be in nature. Listen for its message. I take a walk and see a large tree trunk lying on the ground. From the dried bark I know the tree was cut a while ago, likely due to disease. I lean against the bark feeling the strength of this massive tree. Later, I learn it is a white pine. I spread the blanket I have brought with me and lie beside the tree. I prepare for a journey the way I am used to, travelling to the rock crevice by kayak in my mind.

The eagle is waiting for me. The tree trunk is there. I sense I am to lie on the tree. When I do, I feel the hard edges of bark digging into my back. I become aware of a pull in my chest, like something inside me is being drawn into the tree. The thought startles me and I start to sit up, but I sense that the tree is strong and accepting. I lay back down, knowing that years of sorrow are seeping out of me. After a short time, I feel lighter, like my burden is lifted. Another thought comes to mind: it is no longer necessary to carry the burden of those souls. I have grieved for them long enough.

During the week I embark on many journeys, each one leaving me feeling more connected to the Divine, to an inner truth, to a spirit guide I trust. By the end of the seven days, I feel refreshed and invigorated. I drive home thinking how I almost cancelled out because it all sounded so 'woo-woo'. And yet I feel like I gained so much.

Trauma is multi-faceted. It doesn't just affect the body and mind. It affects the soul as well. To my knowledge, traditional medicine has not found a way to heal the soul. So how do we heal our souls? For those with traditional religious beliefs, spiritual counselling is an option. For others, tapping into the spirit through less conventional ways, may be beneficial. But it is an aspect of healing that shouldn't be disregarded.

Chapter 36

A plethora of scientific studies have documented the incredible benefits of meditation including physiological benefits like decreased blood pressure, improved immune function and decreased inflammatory disorders. Among the many emotional benefits are improved mood, increased empathy and sense of well-being, decreased depression and increased resilience against adversity and the negative effects of stress.

There are hundreds of types of meditation, but generally speaking they all fall into one of two categories. *Focused attention* uses sustained focus on a mantra, an object or an inward focus on the body (such as the breath) to help still the mind. *Open monitoring* is a state of mind where an individual monitors the content of experience from moment to moment. Thoughts or images arise and, without reaction, you take inventory and let them pass. This has always been my preferred method, but I often have to begin the session with several minutes of focusing on the breath as a way to relax and settle.

I was first introduced to meditation through a yoga teacher who guided us through a meditation at the end of each class. Its calming effect had a way of unwinding any tension and stress, and it soon became my favourite part of the class. But like any discipline, being diligent about practicing it on a regular basis makes all the difference in the world.

When I first began to meditate on my own, I had lofty goals of doing so for thirty minutes a day. I planned for times when I was home alone, took the phone off the hook and closed my bedroom door. Initially, I had a lot of difficulty quieting the "monkey brain." Random thoughts would drift into my mind and I tried to still them. Sometimes uncomfortable thoughts bubbled to the surface, making the experience less than pleasant. Sometimes I fell asleep, other times I ended my session feeling that it was useless. In my search to learn as much as I could about mediation, I read books and practiced with CDs using guided imagery. Eventually, I learned to let go of the expectation that I could wipe clear the slate of my mind, and found I was more successful. Some people use mantras as a focal point, others recite prayer beads like the rosary. The style and type of meditation is unique for each individual. One of the most satisfying benefits of meditation is discovering an inner voice, one that may be heard only when the mind is quiet.

The Monroe Institute (TMI), which has been in operation since the mid-seventies, explores, researches and teaches seminars about human consciousness. Through the use of technology known as Hemi-Sync, which utilizes binaural auditory beats to synchronize the brain, participants can experience personal exploration of consciousness, expanded awareness and discovery of self. Intrigued, I sign up for their Gateway Voyage, the prerequisite course in a series of many offered and then marvel at how far I've come at stepping outside my comfort zone, all in an effort to heal.

I choose to take a week-long workshop at one of TMI's satellite sites instead of its Virginia campus, so I fly into San

Francisco and take a shuttle to Petuluma. Nestled in rolling hills, the Institute of Noetic Sciences (IONS) will be hosting our group of fifteen, plus two instructors for the next five days, providing accommodation, meals and meeting rooms. When I arrive, I am assigned a single room in one of the five dormitories, each with eight bedrooms and two common bathrooms. The room has a desk and bureau, and the window overlooks a valley thick with oak trees. Among the amenities here are a labyrinth, sweat lodge, numerous hiking trails and a meditation hut.

Our instructors welcome us into the gathering area where chairs are arranged in a circular fashion. I look around the room; we are a diverse group ranging in age from mid-twenties to sixty-plus. As each of us stands to introduce ourselves, we are encouraged to speak a little about our lives and why we are here. Among us are business executives, an archaeologist, a farmer, a massage therapist, a homemaker and a philosopher. We each come with a curiosity as to what Hemi-Sync will do for our meditative practices.

The instructors waste no time in getting started. We are each given equipment that will pipe binaural beats infused with soft meditative music, which we will listen to with headphones. These meditations are done privately in our rooms, and afterwards we return to the meeting hall to discuss our experiences. It doesn't take long for the group to bond; the nature of our discussions is very personal at times, leaving no room for interpersonal barriers. Over the course of the next five days, we will eat, sleep and meditate. There is a lot of laughter, tears and revelations. A profound sense of goodwill permeates our group. As our sessions continue, we strive for deeper levels of consciousness. All of us agree that the binaural beats seem to accelerate the ability to enter a deeply meditative state.

Close to the end of our workshop, I review the journal entries I made after each meditation. I have written several times about the image of a woman reaching out to me with an outstretched hand. Although a few relatives who have passed on have come to me, this woman I can't place. It is during one of the last sessions that her mystery is revealed to me.

I am in the turret of an ancient building, the stone walls covered in rough plaster. There is no glass on the windows, and a breeze swirls around the room. Off to one side is a spiral staircase leading down. I walk over and peer into the abyss. I am hesitant to descend the stairs since it is dark and I suddenly feel afraid. I take a deep breath and summon the courage. Part way down, the woman beckons me with a kind and inviting smile. I feel a rush of warmth and take a few steps closer. She reaches her hand out to me, and just then I realize who she is. She is my higher self. Her smile broadens as she realizes what I have discovered. Although we aren't communicating with words, our thoughts flow easily between us. I am filled with awe. The warmth she radiates makes me feel that everything is at it should be. All will be well. The music signals a return and I know I must leave her. She places a hand on my shoulder to reassure me that she is always there.

*

As I've mentioned before, the healing of trauma is highly personal. Although the traditional methods of treatment are hugely beneficial, I was determined to explore all types of healing, conventional or otherwise. I wanted to feel like my old self again. Using clues such as the level of excitement I would feel about an approach, many of the methods I chose to guide the healing path were largely intuitive in nature. Exploring different approaches, geared to individual interests can be highly instrumental.

Chapter 37

As so often is the case with STS, relationships suffer. During my most difficult years, instead of reaching out to my husband, family or a friend, I sought refuge in a carefully constructed cocoon. Someone once said to me that if you have one really good friend, you'll never need a therapist. Humans are social by nature, and so isolating ourselves from others can be detrimental to health and well-being. The negative effects include disturbed sleep patterns, increased blood pressure, decreased tolerance to stress and increased risk for depression and suicide.[15] I had been adamant that the move to Winnipeg would be all about healing, and this meant taking steps to repair old relationships and forge new ones.

I meet Cris through hockey. Matt, my younger son, plays on the same team as her son. We get to know each other at the arena while the boys have practices, games or tournaments. We have many common interests, a great starting point for any friendship. Perhaps her most redeeming quality is her patience. She allows our friendship to develop gradually, in a way that never makes me feel overwhelmed. Bit by bit she manages to peel away the threads of my cocoon.

Another quality I love about Cris is her attitude toward self-care. She has become my guru in that respect. She has a deeply rooted understanding of how important self-care is. It has been so energizing to have someone not only validate its importance but to champion my own efforts to incorporate self-care into my life. I have no doubt that if Cris had been around during my most difficult years, things would have turned out differently.

In the fall of 2011, Cris and I take a vacation – an organized Sacred Tour of France, an opportunity to explore a land rich in the tradition of the Divine Feminine. As we roam the south of France with a small group of fellow sojourners, we take in the legends of Mary Magdalene, the Gnostics, the Cathars, the Black Madonnas and the Virgin Mary. Each day holds opportunities for inspiration and profound spiritual connections as we visit sites like the Grotto de la St. Baume where Mary Magdalene is said to have spent the last years of her life, and the natural spring that many believe has curative powers. We tour medieval cities like Carcassone, Minerve, and Montsegur, steeped in Cathar history. In Lourdes, I reconnect with the comfort I experienced with the Virgin Mary, someone I had always turned to as a child. How and why did I lose that connection, I wonder?

At Chartres Cathedral, we walk the labyrinth built into the floor during the thirteenth century. Its circuitous path winds its way to the centre, symbolizing a journey inward. Some people enter a labyrinth with a question or intention. My only hope is to receive insight into my own life. With that thought, I begin a walking meditation. By the time I reach the centre, I feel that I have released enough of my thoughts to be open to new ones. As I stand there, I feel an intense sadness about my relationship with Bill, about how much we have grown apart and how cloudy our future seems. I don't want to think about that. I try to brush the thought away, but it keeps coming back. After I take a few breaths, I get the distinct feeling that I am being told not to give up on what we have. I know the feeling doesn't come from me.

When I return from France, I know I have to face up to things at home. Although I have always cherished my relationship with my husband, it has taken on different faces over the years. During the worst years of my career, we remained partners in life, in parenting and in finances, but our relationship was confined to those areas. Although our life goals aligned, it was as if we were travelling on two separate roads, albeit parallel ones. We had grown apart, and I didn't feel comfortable sharing everything I was going through. The struggles I experienced at work were foreign to Bill. Men and women often see things differently, but that only partly explains my withdrawal. More fundamentally, my detachment from my husband was a symptom of STS. Studies of veterans suffering from PTSD indicate high levels of separation and divorce, two times greater than for veterans without PTSD.

It is time to try to salvage what is left of us, even if that means rehashing old hurts. If I let more time lapse, there might not be anything left to repair.

I am reluctant to broach the subject of our relationship, afraid of the reaction I will get and the unravelling of our comfortable lives, but one day things start spilling out. Although Bill is taken by surprise, he agrees with much of what I am saying. Since he is as committed to doing what it takes as I am, we spend the next few weeks voicing everything we feel we have to, to get back on track. No stone is left unturned, and by the end of those weeks we are emotionally drained but confident that things will work out.

A few months later we head to Banff to celebrate our twenty-fifth wedding anniversary, staying at the same place where we spent our honeymoon. The hotel hasn't changed much, but we have, and we both recognize how fortunate we are. There is nothing like taking stock of what you really value about the other person, remembering why you fell in love in the first place, and falling in love all over again with the people you have become.

After a lovely meal in a restaurant downtown, we head for the hot springs. Although it is below zero, we don our bathing suits and slip into the steamy hot mineral water. Large fluffy snowflakes begin to fall, each one sparkling like the stars that fill the sky. It is magical, and exactly what we need to reconnect. I look over at him, steam rising from the pool, deeply grateful that we have not become another statistic in failed marriages.

Chapter 38

Spending time in nature has a way of grounding you. Even as little as a ten-minute walk around a garden or trail can refocus the mind, release some tension and make you more mindful.

A favourite thing for Bill and me to do is kayaking. Either early in the morning or later in the day, when the water on the lake is as still as glass, we head out along the rocky shores of our cottage on Black Sturgeon Lake in the Kenora area of northern Ontario.

Pristine white, red and jack pines flourish along the shoreline and populate the numerous islands on the lake. Our cottage is on the tip of a peninsula, and so we begin paddling toward the bay that separates our peninsula from the next. Our paddles make little noise, and all we can hear are the frogs, birds and crackle of branches from squirrels on the shore. Ahead, Bill points to a rock in the water that has a turtle on it. As we draw closer, the turtle slips into the lake. We paddle quietly past a loon sitting still on the mud-thatched nest, hoping not to disturb it. It is a pleasant summer evening, with the orange hues of sunset streaking across the sky. Dusk is almost upon us, and the moon is full and round. We head back to the cottage for a bonfire. It has been a perfect day.

The next morning we decide to go for a hike. Bill locks up the shed before we leave. His hollers startle me and I look over to see him swatting away a few hornets. I come closer and see a nest under the eavestrough. I am not sure what has stung him, but I am hoping it is not the black hornets with white facial markings that have already stung us this year. First the dog, then me, then Bill. A sting that feels like an electric current. The pain does not subside for a long while. When Bill was stung, his whole arm swelled up. I swallow hard, knowing that allergies to bee, wasp and hornet stings can worsen with each exposure. Bill has backed away from the nest and is rubbing his neck.

"Bill, get in the car, we're going to emerg." I am trying to calm the panic that is rising in me. My gut screams that this is not good. I don't stop to think that my gut has forsaken me before, so why should I trust it now?

"Let me just spray the bastards. Can you get me the Raid?"

I roll my eyes, knowing he won't come with me until he sprays the nest. I run inside and grab the can. He starts spraying, which sends another flurry of hornets out after him, but he manages to avoid them. Bill throws the can off to the side and looks down.

"Gosh, I don't feel very well." He is blinking and twisting his neck.

I run to the passenger door, open and yell for him to get in. If I call an ambulance, too much time will be lost. "Get in!" I yell in a tone that leaves no doubt.

I begin driving down our road, the gravel spewing up behind us. When I get to the main road, it will take another ten minutes to the hospital.

"Uh, I can't see very well."

I look over at my husband; he is a ghastly shade of white. Then he collapses forward his seatbelt holding him in place but his head bobbing with the bumpiness of the road. Still driving, I reach over to shake him. He is unconscious. He begins to vomit. *Oh God this can't be happening.* I tilt his head down so he doesn't choke. I try to find his carotid pulse but it's impossible. I can't drive and do this. Ahead is an intersection. I have the red light. Just past the lights is an isolated bait and tackle shop. If I can get there, I can pull over and check Bill out. I can call for help. I look both ways and speed through the intersection. I pull into the parking lot, rush around to the passenger side, undo Bill's seatbelt and hoist him from behind, dragging him onto the gravel. His feet are caught in the car, but I have him lying on his side. The fellow working at the bait shop runs out and I tell him to call 911, to tell them he is unconscious, in anaphylactic shock from a bee sting. I sweep Bill's mouth out with my thumb to clear the vomit and feel for a pulse. *Please, not like this.*

Bill's eyes flutter open. "Where are we? Am I on the road?" He spits something from his mouth. He looks down at his shirt, covered in vomit. He looks at me puzzled, "Did I throw up?"

I feel his pulse, steady but slow at around fifty-two beats per minute. I tell him to remain lying, the ambulance is on its way. I tell him how he passed out. By the time the ambulance arrives Bill is coherent, but hives are covering his neck, chest and arms. The paramedics tell me his blood pressure is 78/40. They help him onto the stretcher and I follow the ambulance to the hospital.

Several hours later Bill receives another dose of intravenous glucocorticoid. The initial dose corrected his blood pressure and pulse, but the hives are back with a vengeance. He is covered from head to toe in pink splotchy areas. I sit in a chair beside my husband's stretcher, relieved to relinquish his care to the emergency staff. Our nurse, a young man with a pleasant demeanour, explains everything he is doing, which helps to relieve the anxiety we both feel.

When Bill drifts into sleep, the whole scene plays back in my mind. I breathe, trying to release the adrenalin. As I think back, I am surprised I was able to get my husband out of the car. He is a big strapping lad, and although I am not tiny, there is a huge difference between us. I think back to how he regained consciousness on his own, and then I remember that his legs were caught in the car. Elevation of the legs is often used in the treatment of shock to increase the blood flow to vital organs. His blood pressure and pulse were dangerously low, which is why he passed out. His blood pressure bottomed out. Without any antihistamines, it should not have improved. And yet he came to.

I am shuddering at what a close call it was when I feel the warmth of a flannel blanket around my shoulders. The nurse noticed my shivering and comforts me with this small gesture. As Bill recuperates, I do my best to release my own negative emotions. And then I realize something. This is one of those moments I have feared for so many years: a family member becoming sick and relying on me. Would I have what it took?

I smile. Things turned out okay. Bill will be fine and I kept my wits about me. I shake my head at the journey I have been on in the last ten years. The difficulty in drudging up things that I would much rather have left alone. My perspective and how much I have changed. All the small and seemingly insignificant ways STS has affected me. I am grateful my story didn't end in an inability to help a loved one, in depression, drug addiction or divorce. It did not end in suicide. Now more than ever, I am glad I made the effort to heal.

Afterword

It's been ten years since I left my career behind. And while I started writing almost immediately after I left, it wasn't until the last five years that I knew what I wanted to say. At first, my writing took on the ramblings of a broken nurse. The world as I had known it had shifted. That prompted a journey to discover what was wrong. It was not easy, since secondary traumatic stress was a little known fact back then. The more I learned about STS, the more it all made sense.

Another reason that it took ten years to write the book was the ending. It took that long before I felt I had truly journeyed *through* my experience. I had years of stuff to clear, and the whole idea of self-care was a skill I was learning for the first time. I was determined that my story would have a happy ending, and it does.

During the course of writing this book, terminology has been a challenge. Not unlike the soldier whose diagnosis would change from "shell shock" or "battle fatigue" to eventually post-traumatic stress disorder, we are still very much in the infancy stage of understanding the trauma experienced by people who witness the suffering of others. Is it compassion fatigue? Secondary traumatic stress? Or PTSD? According to Charles

Figley, the terms compassion fatigue and secondary traumatic stress are synonymous. I opted to use secondary traumatic stress for two reasons: first, I was treated for STS, and second, the term compassion fatigue to me implies a loss of compassion, and that is never how I felt. It was more like the compassion I felt had become trapped, and I was paralysed and unable to put it to use.

To further complicate matters, in the last few years the definition for PTSD has undergone some major changes in the DSM-5 (*Diagnostic and Statistical Manual of Mental Disorders*, 5th edition). Those changes can be interpreted to include the emotional trauma of witnessing suffering on a frequent basis. The bottom line is trauma is trauma. The risk factors, the symptoms and the treatments are similar. Seek professional help for a confirmed diagnosis and treatment. Consider additional healing with less conventional forms of treatment if they feel right for you.

Even though STS cost me my career, I consider myself lucky. Recently there has been increased publicity about traumatic stress not just among soldiers of war but among paramedics, firefighters and police. Sadly many of those stories end tragically in suicide. Hopefully, with increased media coverage word will spread. Knowledge is key. There is help out there and access to trained professional help is essential.

Health care practitioners of all disciplines need to understand that trauma and stress-related disorders can happen to them. We will never be able to change the fact that health care professionals witness suffering daily, so we have to change the way we witness it. Resilience training and a commitment to self-care strategies are essential. We must recognize that the burden of caring we feel is not a weakness. Opening this all up to discussion, setting aside the old axiom to "suck it up and carry on" is the only way we will prevent valuable, caring individuals from leaving professions that are in such great demand.

Trauma does not have to be a life sentence, but it will be if steps aren't taken. Anything that robs your life of joy deserves attention. A journey to healing is well worth it. More than that, it can be transformational. I have learned more about myself in the last few years than I did in the forty-plus years before. STS doesn't need to ruin your life; your vision of life can return to technicolour, and not remain sepia forever. You can embrace the joy in small moments, and love with all your heart.

But it is up to you.

Acknowledgments

A heartfelt thanks to my family for their patience and understanding: Bill, thank you for knowing me so well, for believing in me and for filling our lives with laughter. You give me strength and confidence. Mike and Matt, the challenges we face in life often define who we are, I hope this book helps you to understand me better. Thank you for all the life lessons you teach me. You mean the world to me. Mom, your love is inspirational, thank you for showing me by example that spirituality is a gift to hold dear.

Many thanks to both my writers' groups – the Great Pretenders and the Summer Writer's Group – for their constructive feedback and most importantly, their encouragement. I would also like to thank Ellie Barton, my editor, for her keen attention to detail and her insightful comments.

A big hug to Cris for being a true friend. You have been there with me through some very dark times and I will always be grateful. So many of life circumstances become more bearable when you have a friend to lean on.

To Danita, your courage and determination is inspiring. Thank you for the gentle nudge to see this book through to completion and for paving the way by publishing your own book. I am certain that wherever life takes us, we will always remain connected.

I would be amiss in not recognizing the pioneers in research on traumatic disorders, people like Charles Figley, Anna Baranowsky, Peter Levine and Eric Gentry. I hope that in the years to come, we will learn so much more from the work you are doing.

Notes

Chapter 7

1 Charles R. Figley, ed., *Compassion Fatigue: Coping with Secondary Traumatic Stress Disorder in Those Who Treat the Traumatized* (New York: Brunner-Routledge, 1995), 7.

2 Charles R. Figley, ed., *Treating Compassion Fatigue* (New York: Brunner-Routledge, 2002), 19.

Chapter 8

3 S.S. Kim, S. Kaplowitz, and M.V. Johnston, "The Effects of Physician Empathy on Patient Satisfaction and Compliance," *Evaluation and the Health Professions* 3, (September 27, 2004): 237–51, Pubmed: 15312283.

4 Carolyn Zahn-Waxler, Marion Radke-Yarrow, Elizabeth Wagner, and Michael Chapman, "Development of Concern for Others," *Developmental Psychology* 28, no. 1 (1992): 126–36, http://dx.doi.org/10.1037/0012-1649/28/1.126.

5 Elaine N. Aron, *The Highly Sensitive Person: How to Thrive When the World Overwhelms You* (New York: Three Rivers Press, 1998), xiv–37.

Chapter 9

6 Daniel Chen, Robert Lew, Warren Hershman, and Jay Orlander, "A Cross-Sectional Measurement of Medical Student Empathy," *International Journal of General Medicine* 10 (October 22, 2007): 1434–38, http://dx.doi.org/10.1007/s11606-007-0298-x.

7 Hooria Jazaieri, Geshe Thupten Jinpa, Kelly McGonigal, Erika L. Rosenberg, Joel Finkelstein, Emiliana Simon-Thomas, Margaret Cullen, James R. Doty, James J. Gross, and Philippe R. Goldin, "Enhancing Compassion: A Randomized Controlled Trial of a Compassion Cultivation Training Program," *Journal of Happiness Studies* 14, no. 4 (2013): 1113–26, http://dx.doi.org/10.1007%2Fs10902-012-9373-z#/.

Chapter 14

8 Anna B. Baranowsky, "The Silencing Response in Clinical Practice: On the Road to Dialogue," in *Treating Compassion*, ed. Charles R. Figley (New York: Brunner-Routledge, 2002), 155–70.

Chapter 16

9 M. Kingma, "Workplace Violence in the Health Sector: A Problem of Epidemic Proportion," *International Nursing Review* 48, no. 3 (2001): 129–30, http//dx.doi.org//10.1046/j.1466-7657.2001.00094x.

Chapter 18

10 T. Monroe and H. Kenaga, "Don't Ask Don't Tell: Substance Abuse and Addiction among Nurses," *Journal of Clinical Nursing* 20, no. 3-4 (2011): 504–9, Pubmed: 21040041.

Chapter 21

11 Margot Shields and Kathryn Wilkins, *Findings from the 2005 National Survey of the Work and Health of Nurses* (Ottawa: Health Statistics Division, Statistics Canada, 2006), 18. https://secure.cihi.ca/free_products/NHSRep06_ENG.pdf

Chapter 22

12 Gabor Maté, *When the Body Says No: The Cost of Hidden Stress* (Toronto: Knopf, 2003), 7.

13 Heather Stuckey and Jeremy Nobel, "The Connection between Art, Healing and Public Health: A Review of Current Literature," *American Journal of Public Health* 100, no. 2 (2010): 254–63, doi:10.2105/AJPH.2008.156497.

14 Robert Carroll, "Finding the Words to Say It: The Healing Power of Poetry," *Evidence Based Complementary and Alternative Medicine* (Oxford University Press) 2, no. 2 (2005): 164, doi:10.1093/ecam/neh096.

Chapter 35

15 Hara Estroff Marano, "The Dangers of Loneliness," *Psychology Today*, last modified November 20, 2015, http://www.psychologytoday.com/articles/200307/the-dangers-loneliness.

Further Reading

Waking the Tiger: Healing Trauma, by Peter Levine and Ann Frederick (Berkeley, California: North Atlantic Books, 1997)

Man's Search for Meaning, by Viktor E. Frankl (Boston: Beacon Press, 2006)

Emotional Freedom: Liberate Yourself from Negative Emotions and Transform Your Life, by Judith Orloff, MD. (New York: Random House, 2009)

On Grief and Grieving: Finding the Meaning of Grief Through the Five Stages of Loss, by Elizabeth Kubler-Ross and David Kessler (New York: Simon and Schuster, 2005)

The Art of Healing: Uncovering Your Inner Wisdom and Potential for Self Healing, by Bernie S. Siegel (California: New World Library, 2013)

Online self-test for Secondary Traumatic Stress: www.proqol.org